Kleinian Theory

A contemporary perspective

Kleinian Theory

A contemporary perspective

Edited by
CATALINA BRONSTEIN

Member of the British Psycho-Analytical Society and Honorary
Senior Lecturer, University College London

W

WHURR PUBLISHERS

LONDON AND PHILADELPHIA

© 2001 Whurr Publishers
First published 2001 by
Whurr Publishers Ltd
19B Compton Terrace, London N1 2UN, England and
325 Chestnut Street, Philadelphia PA 19106, USA

Reprinted 2002, 2003, 2006 and 2007

British Library Cataloguing in Publication Data
A catalogue record for this book is available from the British
Library.

ISBN-13: 978 1 86156 226 5 p/b

Contents

Series foreword

After the first hundred years of its history, psychoanalysis has matured into a serious, independent intellectual tradition, which has notably retained its capacity to challenge established truths in most areas of our culture. The biological psychiatrist of today is called to task by psychoanalysis, as much as was the specialist in nervous diseases of Freud's time, in turn of the century Vienna. Today's cultural commentators, whether for or against psychoanalytic ideas, are forced to pay attention to considerations of unconscious motivation, defences, early childhood experience and the myriad other discoveries which psychoanalysts brought to 20th century culture. Above all, psychoanalytic ideas have spawned an approach to the treatment of mental disorders, psychodynamic psychotherapy, which has become the dominant tradition in most countries, at least in the Western world.

Little wonder that psychoanalytic thinking continues to face detractors, individuals who dispute its epistemology and its conceptual and clinical claims. While disappointing in one way, this is a sign that psychoanalysis may be unique in its capacity to challenge and provoke. Why should this be? Psychoanalysis is unrivalled in the depth of its questioning of human motivation, and whether its answers are right or wrong, the epistemology of psychoanalysis allows it to confront the most difficult problems of human experience. Paradoxically, our new understanding concerning the physical basis of our existence - our genes, nervous systems and endocrine functioning – rather than finally displacing psychoanalysis, has created a pressing need for a complementary discipline which considers the memories, desires and meanings which are beginning to be recognised as influencing human adaptation even at the biological level. How else, other than through the study of subjective experience, will we understand the expression of the individual's biological destiny, within the social environment?

It is not surprising, then, that psychoanalysis continues to attract some of the liveliest intellects in our culture. These individuals are by no means all psychoanalytic clinicians, or psychotherapists. They are distinguished scholars in an almost bewildering range of disciplines, from the study of mental disorders with their biological determinants to the disciplines of literature, art, philosophy and history. There will always be a need to explicate the meaning of experience. Psychoanalysis, with its commitment to understanding subjectivity, is in a premier position to fulfil this intellectual and human task. We are not surprised at the upsurge of interest in psychoanalytic studies in universities in many countries. The books in this series are aimed at addressing the same intellectual curiosity that has made these educational projects so successful.

We are proud that the Whurr Series in Psychoanalysis has been able to attract some of the most interesting and creative minds in the field. Our commitment is to no specific orientation, to no particular professional group, but to the intellectual challenge to explore the questions of meaning and interpretation systematically, and in a scholarly way. Nevertheless, we would be glad if this series particularly spoke to the psychotherapeutic community, to those individuals who use their own minds and humanity to help others in distress.

Our focus in this series is to communicate the intellectual excitement which we feel about the past, present and future of psychoanalytic ideas. We hope that our work with the authors and editors in the series will help to make these ideas accessible to an ever-increasing and worldwide group of students, scholars and practitioners.

Peter Fonagy
Mary Target
University College London
October 2000

Acknowledgements

I would like to acknowledge my gratitude to Peter Fonagy and Mary Target for their encouragement to carry out the project of editing this book. I am also indebted to the students of the Master course at the Psychoanalysis Unit, University College London, whose comments, doubts and interest in Melanie Klein's work stimulated the wish to refine the teaching of psychoanalytic concepts.

I would like to thank the Melanie Klein Trust for their kind permission to reproduce unpublished material from the Klein Archives held at the Wellcome Institute for the History of Medicine.

A number of people have helped with the editorial work. I am greatly indebted to Mary Target for her helpful comments on the manuscript. I am also grateful to Elizabeth Allison for her help with the references and to Julian Target for his help with the editing of some of the chapters.

I am deeply indebted to Elizabeth Bott Spillius for her extremely valuable suggestions on the manuscript as well as for her unlimited patience in answering the numerous questions that arose during the editing of this book.

Finally, I wish to express my gratitude to my family for their support and understanding of the time taken away from them.

List of contributors

David Bell is a member of the British Psycho-Analytical Society and Consultant Psychiatrist in Psychotherapy at the Tavistock Clinic London. He teaches Freud at the Institute of P-A and lectures on the University College Masters Programme. He has written various papers and chapters in books and is editor of *Reason and Passion* and *Culture and Psychoanalysis: a Kleinian perspective*.

Jill Boswell grew up in South Africa, and holds a degree in English Literature from the University of Cape Town. She moved to London in 1965, and became a marriage counsellor and then a psychotherapist before training at the Institute of Psycho-Analysis. She is now in private practice. She has a particular interest in the interplay of insight between psychoanalysis and literature.

Ronald Britton, FRC PSYCH. is known internationally as a psychoanalytic writer and teacher. His books include *The Oedipus Complex Today* and *Belief and Imagination* which includes, in addition to clinical papers, studies on Wordsworth, Rilke, Milton and Blake. He was educated at Lancaster Royal Grammar School and University College London and in the 1970s was Chair of the Dept. for Children and Families, Tavistock Clinic London. Currently he is a Training Analyst of the British Psycho-Analytical Society and a member of the Board of the Melanie Klein Trust. He is married and has three children and five grandchildren.

Catalina Bronstein (née Halperin) is a Training and Supervising Analyst of the British Institute of Psycho-Analysis and a member of the Association of Child Psychotherapists. She studied medicine and qualified as a psychiatrist in Buenos Aires, Argentina. She trained as a child psychotherapist at the Tavistock Clinic and as an analyst at the British Institute of Psycho-Analysis. For the last twelve years she has been working at the Brent Adolescent Centre and in private practice. She is Honorary Senior Lecturer in Psychoanalytic Theory at University College London and teaches at the Tavistock Clinic and abroad. Currently, she is Associate Editor of the New Library of Psychoanalysis.

Marco Chiesa is Consultant Psychiatrist in Psychotherapy and Head of the Research Unit at the Cassel Hospital, Richmond; he is also Honorary Senior Lecturer at University College London. Formerly he was Senior Clinical Tutor in Psychotherapy at the Institute of Psychiatry (London) and Hon. Consultant Psychotherapist at the Maudsley and Bethlem NHS Mental Health Trust (London). He is a full member of the British Psycho-Analytical Society and is engaged in private psychoanalytical practice.

Betty Joseph is a Member of the British Psycho-Analytical Society. She is a Training Analyst supervising both child and adult cases. Her training analyst was Michael Balint, but subsequently being particularly interested in the work of Melanie Klein she had further analysis with Paula Heimann. She has travelled extensively in Europe, North and South America, Australia, India, Israel etc. lecturing, participating in conferences and doing clinical seminars and supervisions. In 1995 she was awarded a Mary Sigourney Award in New York for outstanding contributions to psychoanalysis. In 1989 a collection of her papers was published by Routledge, edited by Elizabeth Bott Spillius and Michael Feldman entitled *Psychic Equilibrium and Psychic Change*. Her main interest in psychoanalysis has always been primarily in the clinical and technical aspects.

Ruth Riesenberg-Malcolm is a Training and Supervising Analyst of the British Psycho-Analytical Society. She qualified as a Psychoanalyst in Chile, coming to London for further training. She formerly created and organized the Department of Social Work and a Therapeutic Community in the University of Chile Medical School Psychiatric Clinic. Later at the same clinic she developed the child psychology and child analysis service. She is in full-time private psychoanalytic practice. In 1999 she published a book entitled *On Bearing Unbearable States of Mind*.

Priscilla Roth is a Training and Supervising Analyst at the British Psycho-Analytical Society. She is a graduate in psychology of the University of California at Berkeley and did research into mental illness in California and Massachusetts before training as a child and adolescent psychotherapist at the Tavistock Institute, London, and then as a psychoanalyst at the British Institute of Psycho-Analysis. She is currently a Senior Psychotherapist in the Adolescent Department of the Tavistock Clinic. She teaches at the Institute of Psycho-Analysis, the Tavistock Clinic, the University of London Psychoanalytic Theory course, and abroad.

Hanna Segal was born in Poland in 1918. Her secondary education was partly in Poland and partly in Geneva. She started studying medicine in Warsaw in 1937 and after the war qualified in Edinburgh in 1946. She then moved to London where she entered psychoanalytic training in 1947. Her training analyst was Melanie Klein and her first supervisors were Joan Riviere and Paula Heinman. She has been President of the British Psycho-Analytical Society twice and Vice-President of the IPA. She has also been a founding Fellow of the Royal College of Psychiatry and of Psychoanalysts for the Prevention of Nuclear War (British) (PPNW) and International Psychoanalysts Against Nuclear Weapons (IPANW). She is the author of several articles, mainly in the IPGA, and of five books. She is a widow with three children and four grandchildren.

Elizabeth Bott Spillius was born in Canada, studied psychology as an undergraduate and then social anthropology at the University of Chicago and the London School of Economics. She published an anthropological study of London families called *Family and Social Network* in 1957 and later a monograph on the Kingdom of Tonga. She was trained in psycho-analysis at the Institute of Psycho-Analysis in London, is a Training Analyst and works in private practice. She has published several papers and edited a two-volume book, *Melanie Klein Today*. She was Editor of Books for the Institute of Psycho-Analysis for 10 years.

Jane Temperley: after a BA in Modern History from Oxford University (St Anne's College), she studied social work at Bristol University and obtained a Masters Degree in Social Work from the University of Connecticut. She worked as a psychiatric social worker at St Mary's Hospital Paddington and then at the Tavistock Clinic, where she became Principal Social Worker in the Adult Department. She qualified as a psychoanalyst in 1975 and is a Member of the British Psycho-Analytical Society now working in private practice. She lectures at University College London.

Introduction

CATALINA BRONSTEIN

The aim of this book is to present an account of the main theoretical concepts in Kleinian theory as they have been postulated by Melanie Klein, together with newer developments and formulations inspired by her work.

This book was developed from the experience of teaching Kleinian theory to students of the MSc Course on Theoretical Psychoanalytic Studies at University College London. Many works have already been published, about Klein or her theories (see for example Baranger, 1971; Grosskurth, 1986; Hinshelwood, 1989; Kristeva, 2000; Meltzer, 1978; Mitchell, 1991; Petot, 1979, 1982; Segal, 1973, 1979; Spillius, 1994; Schafer, 1997, to name but a few), but it was felt that there was a need for a clear and comprehensible exposition of Kleinian thinking that would include both Klein's ideas and the main developments that have arisen from them and that would be accessible both to clinicians and to those who come from other academic fields and whose interest in psychoanalysis is mainly academic.

Reading Melanie Klein's work is not always easy. She often wrote using very concrete language, which she felt best expressed the unconscious phantasized world of the infant. As is often the case in the History of Ideas, there are times when a concept may carry different meanings, which is likely to confuse the reader who is just beginning to approach the subject. Klein's ideas are always intimately linked to her clinical experience, theory and practice feeding each other from the very beginning of her career. Her descriptions are mostly closely based on her clinical material. This undoubtedly contributes to the depth of her thinking though it presents some difficulty to those readers who are interested in her theories but who are not clinicians. This book has been written bearing these issues in mind. Even though the chapters have been written in different styles and from different perspectives and there are some inevitable repetitions, it is hoped that this will add to the richness of the presentation without losing its central aim.

Even though Klein saw herself as following in Freud's footsteps, she was also an innovator who introduced a radical change in the way of thinking about the internal world of the child, in the conceptualization of the role of anxiety, unconscious phantasy and internalized objects, as well as in the technique of child analysis. Fundamentally, she developed a clinical approach and new ideas leading to a rich combination of object relations and drive theory. She and her colleagues also opened the door to new ways of approaching mental illness, extending the possibility of providing psychoanalytical help to very young children and to psychotic patients

This book looks at the development of the main concepts in Kleinian theory, starting with a brief biographical description and with the discovery of the psychoanalytic play-technique, which Klein regarded as the equivalent to free association in the adult. Her first discoveries, such as of an early Oedipus Complex, an archaic and very severe superego and the reality of transference in the analysis of young children paved the way for future new findings. Klein's background, the beginnings of her career, her first psychoanalytical postulations, and the influence that her two analysts, Ferenczi and Abraham, had on her work will be discussed in Chapter 1.

Klein moved permanently to England in September 1926, after the death of her analyst, Karl Abraham. She had experienced being ostracized in the Berlin Psychoanalytic Society and her ideas had not been welcomed by the Viennese analysts. However, in England she found a group of analysts eager to listen and to support her, among them Ernest Jones, Susan Isaacs and Joan Riviere. This offered her the possibility to go on developing her ideas on child analysis. In the late 1930s the expansion of fascism and anti-semitism on the Continent mobilized analysts in America and in England to come to the rescue of those colleagues who were at risk. Ernest Jones, with the help of Princess Marie Bonaparte and the American Ambassador in Paris, negotiated with the Nazis for Freud, his family and some of his colleagues to be allowed to leave Austria. This meant that conflict about different approaches to the understanding of psychoanalysis, and in particular of child analysis, which had already existed between the Viennese and the British analysts, had now to be negotiated within one society. The view, which had up to then been accepted in British Psycho-Analytical Society, that Melanie Klein had made a very valuable contribution to child analysis, was not shared by Anna Freud and most of the Viennese colleagues (King and Steiner, 1991). Between 1941 and 1945, disagreement with Kleinian theories as well as emerging political issues led to a series of scientific discussions on controversial issues, now known as the 'Controversial Discussions' (King and Steiner, 1991). It was then that Susan Isaacs produced her paper on 'The nature and function of phantasy' (1943). For Klein, unconscious phantasies *are* the primary unconscious content rather than a transformation, or a disguised form of a primary unconscious content. This basic mental activity is present in rudimentary form from birth onwards. Spillius (Chapter 2) explores this development as well as the differences from Freud's concept of fantasy.

In her work with children, Melanie Klein became quite convinced of the importance of innate aggression. She was the major follower of Freud to adopt his theory of the death drive. The fundamental conflict between the life and death drives, between love and hate, is the deepest source of ambivalence, anxiety and guilt. The infant's impulses to love and hate are present from the very beginning, experienced in terms of his unconscious phantasies about his relationships to his objects.

Klein developed the concept of 'positions' to account for modes of psychic functioning which last throughout life (and are therefore different from Freud's concept of 'stages'). Each of the positions refers to the child's experience of his objects, with the accompanying anxieties about the conflict between his impulses and the defences that his ego institutes against them. The use of the word 'object' rather than 'mother' or 'father' describes who (or what) the infant is relating to in his Unconscious. For example, it may be a 'part' of the mother, such as her breast, her eyes, or even a combination of aspects of both parents, as well as the 'mother'.

Klein's description of the depressive position was chronologically earlier (first described in 1935 and 1940) than that of the paranoid-schizoid position (first described in 1946). For reasons of clarity we have reversed this order and followed instead the order in which Klein believed they develop in the infant, though the oscillations between the two positions continue throughout life.

Chapter 3 on the paranoid-schizoid position illustrates the struggle operating from the beginning of life between the life and the death drives, and the first mechanisms of defence to which the ego resorts: splitting, projection and introjection. Roth describes the early relationship the infant establishes with 'part' objects, how he divides his world by splitting the ego and the object into 'good' and 'bad' in order to protect his sense of his good object – upon which his growing sense of himself depends – from the danger of fragmentation and annihilation. The aim of the ego is to introject and identify with an ideal object to protect itself from the persecutors containing, in phantasy, the projected destructive impulses. This chapter also explores the problems that may arise in the achievement of this healthy bi-polarity.

In the depressive position the infant moves towards a gradual integration of both the ego and the object. Temperley (Chapter 4) explains how the internalization of good experiences with good objects makes the infant feel less threatened and more whole, with a more pronounced sense of separateness. The child becomes aware that he cannot control or possess the object but needs it and misses it. He is able to experience ambivalence as well as anxiety and concern about the state of the mother who is now both hated and loved. The desire to repair and restore the object is beautifully illustrated in the examples presented by Temperley.

Britton (Chapter 5) expands the theory of the two positions (paranoid-schizoid or 'Ps' and depressive or 'D') as it has been developed by Klein. He suggests a model which makes a distinction between developmental and pathological movement. He follows Bion's suggestion that the two positions (Ps and D) alternate throughout life and sees this fluctuation as a continuous life-long cycle of development. This chapter addresses the distinction between a positive psychic development that produces turmoil but that is necessary for change to take place and a pathological regression that reverses development and becomes a retreat into a pathological organization, as described by Steiner (1993), which just reiterates the past and evades future development.

In her work with very young children via the use of the psychoanalytical play technique, Klein came to see that the infant's world can contain primitive oedipal phantasies of a sadistic quality. She also came across early phantasies which made her believe that the child has an innate awareness of the differences between the sexes, for example, of the existence of the vagina in the little girl. Klein places great importance on the early role that the relationship to the mother plays in the sexual development of both boys and girls. In Chapter 6 on the Oedipus Complex, Boswell explores the development of Klein's thinking about the Oedipus Complex, its difference from Freud's ideas as well as the link Klein establishes between the Oedipus Complex and curiosity, learning and symbolizing. She further explores the changes in Klein's early ideas once she developed the concept of the depressive position.

The important role that envy plays in the psychic world of the child has always been present in Klein's theory; for example in her theorizing about the girl's envy of her mother's body (Klein, 1945). But it was mainly in her later work that she singled out envy as one of the most fundamental universal emotions. Envy of the breast can be stirred by gratification (proof of the goodness and richness of the object) as well as by frustration and deprivation. Envy is one of the most painful emotions we have to contend with in that it attacks the goodness of the object, thereby precluding the internalization of a good object and the fostering of the loving and lovable aspects of the self. Envious attacks can give rise to intense guilt, hopelessness and the need to resort to manic defences. Chiesa (Chapter 7) explores the development of this concept in Kleinian theory. Klein's theory of envy became highly controversial. She was accused of focusing excessively on these more destructive and hostile aspects of the self and of giving more importance to the idea of innate aggression than to the reactive aspects of aggression. However, Klein sees the capacity to love as also primitive and existing from the beginning of life and she attributes great importance to the role played by gratitude and the wish to repair the damage done to one's objects.

The concept of 'internal objects', like that of 'unconscious phantasy', is ubiquitous in Klein's theory and it has been described by Segal as 'almost the totality of our emotional experience' (Segal, 1999, p. 96). Even though this concept was present in Freud's work, it was Melanie Klein who developed it further and made it central to her theory of the mind. Freud's and Abraham's studies of melancholia greatly influenced Klein who took up the idea that identification with objects affects the structure of the ego. Chapter 8 ('What are internal objects?') focuses on the development of this concept in Klein, following the path opened up by Freud, Ferenczi and Abraham with their discovery of the mechanisms of projection and introjection. In Klein's view, the primal 'good' object forms the core of the ego (Klein, 1957) as she sees the ego developing round it. But internalized objects can adopt in phantasy any form, and they have been used to convey different experiences in the infant, which range from the very early, pre-verbal and concrete bodily experiences to more sophisticated ones; they could be 'part-objects' as well as 'whole' objects. Their fate is therefore crucially related to whether we are describing them in the context of the paranoid schizoid position or of the depressive position. This concept cannot be thought of in isolation: it is always part of the interaction between other main hypotheses, such as the existence of the life and death drives, the hypothesis of unconscious phantasies and the theory of the two positions, Ps and D.

The concepts of splitting and projective identification are vital to the development of the ego. In 1946 Klein published 'Notes on some schizoid mechanisms' in which she articulated the main anxieties and defences that constitute the paranoid-schizoid position with the recognition that both the object and the ego are altered by them. She there referred to the weakening and impoverishment of the ego resulting from excessive splitting and project-ive identification. The mechanism of projective identification has been thoroughly studied by a number of post-Kleinian analysts and is seen to be central to the understanding of mental phenomena. Bell (Chapter 9) explores how this concept became part of Klein's thinking, starting with Freud's use of the concepts of 'projection' and 'identification'. 'Projective identification' describes at the same time a psychological mechanism of defence, typical of the paranoid-schizoid position, which has a real effect on the state of the ego, and a particular type of unconscious phantasy in which the object is affected by the subject's projections. Bell explores the effect this may have upon the subject as well as on the recipient of these projections. The use of this term is nowadays quite extensive and can describe normal phenomena, such as the early process of communication between mother and infant as well as evacuatory processes which may underlie psychotic states. This chapter describes the contributions made on this subject by Bion, Rosenfeld, Sandler, Segal and Spillius amongst other psychoanalysts.

In Chapter 10 ('Symbolization'), Segal proposes that the understanding of unconscious symbolism is the key to the understanding of all unconscious communication. While Freud and Jones considered that it is the libidinal link which enables symbolization to take place, Klein added the major role played by anxiety in symbol-formation. Through the analysis of an autistic child Klein deduced that the whole process of symbolization came to a stop as a result of his intense anxiety caused by his sadistic phantasized attacks on his mother's body. When, during the analysis, his unconscious anxiety diminished, the child began to speak, play and form relationships. Segal suggests that symbol formation develops gradually from the paranoid-schizoid to a depressive level of functioning. She identifies a phenomenon called 'symbolic equation' where symbols are formed by projective identification and are used to deny any separateness between the subject and the object. This is different from 'true symbolism' in the depressive position, when the object can be given up and mourned, and the role of the father and the parental couple is accepted. The symbol here 'represents' the object rather than being 'equated' to it. Segal's ideas are brought together in this chapter with Bion's theory of thinking and his introduction of the concept of alpha function.

Symbol formation, the role of unconscious phantasies and internal objects and the structure of the ego are explored by Segal in Chapter 11 ('Changing models of the mind') where she looks at the differences between the models of the mind in Freud and Klein and proposes her own way of understanding the way the mind is structured. The exploration of the dialectic relationship between function and structure has been greatly enriched by the ideas developed by Bion in his theory of thinking and of the psychotic aspects of the personality.

Bion's contributions are mentioned in many of this book's chapters. It seemed however important to dedicate a chapter solely to his theory of containment. Riesenberg-Malcolm (Chapter 12) understands this to be an active process by which the infant and the mother are involved in an emotional relationship in which the mother does something akin to 'mental digestion', which the baby cannot do for himself. The baby's fears are dealt with by being projected into the 'good breast' where they are made tolerable and can then be re-introjected. The mother's capacity for reverie develops on both the emotional and on the intellectual level, as her understanding of her baby's needs helps him to discover them. Riesenberg-Malcolm also explores Bion's theory of thinking and his theory of knowledge, both seen as essential contributions to post-Kleinian developments.

The concept of transference is central to psychoanalysis. It therefore seemed pertinent to conclude with a last chapter which could encompass many of the concepts explored throughout the book, concepts which come together as part of the phenomenon of transference. Joseph (Chapter 13) builds on from Klein's description of transference as a 'total situation' transferred from the past into the present. This means not only the picture the patient has of his objects and how his internal world has been constructed, but also how these mechanisms (such as introjection and projective identification) continue operating throughout life, and similarly in the relationship with the analyst. The meaning of transference is not derived just from the patient's past but from his inner world. For Joseph, the concept of transference 'entails a technique by which from the whole material presented the unconscious elements of the transference are deduced'. Joseph explores the importance of following the patient's shifts and changes in his impulses, emotions and defences and the fundamental role of interpretation in promoting psychic change.

Melanie Klein's ideas had a profound impact both on British and international psychoanalysis. Many of her followers continued to develop her theories into what is today a very rich, always expanding school of thought. This reaches not only clinical psychoanalysis but also the academic field (Stonebridge and Phillips, 1998). The impact of Kleinian thinking has expanded well beyond England, into the rest of Europe, South America and Australia. There is a renewed interest in her work in North and Central America and in Asia. Clinical work and writings following her line of thinking are vast. It is hoped that this book will introduce the reader to the work of one great creative thinker and make more available the work of those who continued to develop her ideas.

CHAPTER 1

Melanie Klein: beginnings

CATALINA BRONSTEIN

> It is the attitude, the inner conviction which finds the necessary technique (Klein, 1927, p. 142)

Melanie Klein's ideas developed over many years of working with children and adults. The innovative quality of her thinking and the richness of her ideas were rooted in her early work with children. It is therefore important to examine this first phase of the development of her theories, as it laid the foundations for her later work, and led to the discovery of psychoanalytic play-technique. This first period culminated in the publication of *The Psychoanalysis of Children* (Klein, 1932).

Biographical background

Melanie Klein (née Reizes) was born on 30 March 1882 in Vienna. She was the youngest of four children. The eldest child was a girl called Emilie (born in 1876); a brother, Emanuel, was born in 1877. A second sister, Sidonie, was born in 1878. Melanie Klein's father, Moriz Reizes, came from a rigidly orthodox Jewish family. He had broken away from his orthodox background and had studied in secret, hiding study materials under his Talmud books in order to obtain the German *matura* that enabled him to go to medical school. He was married off to a girl whom he had never met and whom he later divorced. At the age of 44 he fell in love with a 25-year-old woman, Libussa Deutsch, Melanie's mother, whom he married. They settled down in a small town called Deutsch-Kreutz about seventy miles from Vienna. At first, Reizes worked in general practice, but on moving to Vienna the opportunities for professional success as a doctor became rather thin and he was forced to take on a dental practice. Their financial difficulties compelled Libussa to open a shop (she sold plants and reptiles), an unusual thing for a doctor's wife in those days.

Melanie had a liberal upbringing, with religion playing little part in her family life. Melanie herself was an atheist, though very aware of her Jewish roots (Segal, 1979). She was very attracted by the cultural ambience of Libussa's family (Grosskurth, 1986) which she described as containing 'a burning need for knowledge' (Klein, 1959a).

Two of her siblings died young. They both seem to have had a long-lasting and important influence on their sister. Sidonie, four years older than Melanie, developed scrofula; it seems she was ill for one or two years until her death in 1886, when Melanie was four years old. Sidonie told Melanie that she wanted to pass on to her everything she knew before dying, and taught her the principles of counting and reading (Klein, 1959a; Segal, 1979). The relationship with her brother Emanuel also marked her deeply. He was a very musical, artistically gifted boy. From when Melanie was nine and he was impressed by a poem she wrote, Emanuel became her confidant, her friend and teacher and took great interest in her development. Her relationship to Emanuel was a most important factor in her development. Melanie planned to study medicine, and thought of becoming a psychiatrist. Emanuel coached her in Greek and Latin so she could enter the gymnasium. Emanuel was quite a sickly young man who had suffered scarlet fever at 12, followed by tuberculosis and rheumatic fever. Always aware of the possibility of dying young, he did die at the age of 25. Her brother's illness and early death left Melanie with a profound sense of grief:

> Here again I have the feeling that, had one known more about medicine, one might have been able to do something to keep him alive longer, but I have been told that even now rheumatic heart diseases are not always curable. I don't know whether this is true or not, but it left me with the same feeling that I had about my little sister, that many things could have been done to prevent his illness and early death. ... In my memory he remains a young, strong minded man, as I knew him, strong in his opinions, not minding if they were unpopular, with a deep understanding of art and a passion for it in many ways, and the best friend I ever had. (Klein, 1959a)

At the age of 17 Melanie met her future husband, Arthur Klein, a chemical engineering student from the Slovak part of Hungary. She was very much impressed by his intellectual capacity though later felt that she had been influenced by her brother's good opinion of him. She married him in March 1903, at the age of 21, while still mourning the death of Emanuel in December 1902. Her early engagement, marriage and subsequent move prevented Melanie from following the career she had planned. Instead, she went to extramural classes in art and history. The couple settled in Rosenberg in the then Hungarian province of Liptau. They had three children: Melitta, born in 1904, Hans, born in 1907 and Erich, born in 1914. Melanie Klein was quite unhappy there and suffered from bouts of depression. When, in 1909, Arthur was transferred to a small town in Silesia, it was decided that Melanie, her mother and the children, would settle in Budapest. Her mother died there in November 1914. It was during this year that Klein read Freud's 1900 paper on dreams and became interested in psychoanalysis. This was followed by her starting her first personal analysis, with Ferenczi:

> While living in Budapest I had become interested in psycho-analysis. I remember that the first book of Freud's that I read was the small book on Dreams and, when I read it, I knew that that was it – that was what I was aiming at, at least during those years when I was so very keen to find what would satisfy me intellectually and emotionally. I went into analysis with Ferenczi, who was the most outstanding Hungarian analyst, and he very much encouraged my idea of devoting myself to analysis, particularly child analysis, for which he said I had a particular talent. (Klein 1959a)

Ferenczi had an important influence on Melanie Klein's ideas, though apparently of less significance than her second psychoanalyst, Abraham. In 1913 Ferenczi wrote his paper 'Stages in the development of the sense of reality' (Ferenczi S, 1913), where he explored the characteristics of infantile omnipotence and the infant's access to a sense of reality. In this work, he linked infantile omnipotence to what he had previously called the 'introjection phase' in 1909, contrasted with a 'reality stage' which he linked with projection. These concepts were taken up, though later modified, by Melanie Klein. In relation to her own analysis, Klein later questioned Ferenczi for not taking up the negative transference:

> Technique at that time was extremely different from what it is at present and the analysis of negative transference did not enter. I had a very strong positive transference and I feel that one should not underrate the effect of that, though as we know, it can never do the whole job. (Klein, 1959a)

After reading her paper 'The development of a child' (Klein, 1921, Part I) to the Hungarian Psychoanalytical Society, Klein became a member in 1919. By this time, the political situation – derived from the defeat of the Austro-Hungarian Empire, with Bela Kun's invasion of Slovakia and the subsequent Rumanian intervention – contributed to the spread of anti-semitism, affecting many Jewish professionals. Arthur Klein could not continue with his job and left for Sweden where he settled, while Melanie went to live for a year in Slovakia with her parents-in-law. This preliminary separation between husband and wife lasted until 1922 when the couple divorced.

In 1920 Melanie Klein attended the first postwar International Congress of Psychoanalysis in The Hague. It was at this Congress that she first met Hermine Hug-Hellmuth who was already exploring the field of psychoanalysis and education in children. She felt discouraged by the reception that the older analyst gave her. At that Congress she also met Abraham who encouraged her to settle in Berlin.

> In 1920 at the Congress at The Hague, Abraham strongly encouraged me to settle in Berlin and to devote myself to child analysis, and promised me his support, a promise which, like many others he made, he fully kept. (Klein, 1959a).

Klein arrived in Berlin in 1921 at the age of 38, and established a mixed practice, with both adults and children. She approached Abraham with a request for a personal analysis; he at first rejected her request as he was not happy at analysing colleagues but finally accepted her as a patient. Klein started her analysis at the beginning of 1924. Her analysis only lasted nine months as it was ended by Abraham's serious illness in the summer of 1925. This was followed by his premature death at Christmas of that year.

Abraham exercised a very important influence on Melanie Klein. He greatly supported and encouraged her to go on working with children, at times helping her to take very important steps:

> So I worked on my own in Berlin and I only remember one important occasion on which I asked Abraham's advice. That was when the anxiety in the child, whose analysis was the first I mentioned, grew in a way which frightened me. Abraham more or less advised me to go on, some quite important changes in the child had happened and it turned out that I had been at a climax and that a few days later the anxiety went down again. This experience has been definite in developing my methods of approach. I knew now that it was anxiety that one had to analyse, and that, if one could find the unconscious reasons for it, with all the implications, one could diminish it. (Klein, 1959a)

On 22 and 23 April 1924, Klein took part in the Salzburg International Congress where she read a paper 'The technique of the analysis of young children'. This paper, which was never published, formed the first version of her 1926 paper 'The psychological principles of early analysis' (Klein, 1926). Her work made a strong impact on Ernest Jones who invited her to give a series of lectures in London. Other English psychoanalysts, Joan Riviere and Alix Strachey, also became very interested in her work. Klein visited England in July 1925 during an interruption of her own analysis due to Abraham's illness. She was warmly welcomed and Ernest Jones invited her to stay in England at least for a year. Klein returned to Berlin to resume her analysis with Abraham, but his illness, first thought to be bronchitis, was in fact a more serious injury of the pharynx which developed into a pulmonary abscess and finally a subphrenic abscess which caused his death (Petot, 1990).

Abraham's unexpected death was extremely painful to Klein and affected her deeply, both personally and professionally. He had been her main supporter in the Berlin Psycho-Analytical Society, and his death left her isolated. Her work was considered 'unorthodox' by her colleagues, as the Berlin Society followed Anna Freud's views of child analysis (Segal, 1979, p. 33). After Abraham's death, Klein decided to accept Ernest Jones' invitation and finally settled down in England in 1926, where she remained until her own death on 22 September 1960.

Repression, sublimation and the desire for knowledge

The presentation Klein made to the Hungarian Society in 1919 described her views on education and her educational attempts to protect a child from 'over-strong repression' (Klein, 1921). The boy, whom she called Fritz, is thought to have been Klein's own son Erich (Grosskurth, 1986, p. 75). Today it would be considered both strange and undesirable for parents to carry out the analysis of their own children, but at that time it seemed an obvious thing to do. Another example of this was the analysis of 'Little Hans', also carried out by one of his parents (his father) under Freud's direction.

Klein's contention at this time was that sexual enlightenment could protect the child from 'over-strong repression' so preventing future mental illness. Her idea was to provide as much sexual information as 'the growth of his desire for knowledge requires' (Klein, 1921, p. 1). At this point Klein believed that sexual enlightenment would deprive sexuality of its mystery and danger, lessening the need to repress wishes, thoughts and feelings, and therefore exercising a decisive influence upon the development of the child's intellectual capacities.

At that time psychoanalysis postulated that repression of sexuality (mainly of child sexuality) could lead to neurosis. Fritz was subject to certain intellectual inhibitions. He was behind other children of his age in practical matters, and Klein thought that, though intelligent, he was showing a slow pace of mental development. He also displayed marked feelings of omnipotence in conflict with his reality-sense. Klein advocated that honesty and frank answers to all the questions that the child formulates regarding sexuality (as well as life/death issues) could guard against the tendency to repression, which was seen as the chief danger affecting thought. The theory behind this was that a diminution of repression fosters sublimation (Klein, 1921).

Sublimation was described at this time as the capacity to employ 'superfluous libido in a cathexis of ego-tendencies' (Klein, 1923b, p. 81). Repression would act upon these ego-tendencies causing inhibitions. At this first stage Klein felt that the capacity to remain healthy was directly linked to the development of the possibility for sublimation at a very early stage of ego-development (Klein, 1923b). She also thought that the conflict between sexual curiosity and the tendency to repression played a part in the conflict between omnipotence of thought (pleasure principle) and the reality principle, in that the combination of sexual and intellectual interests enabled them to become stronger than the attachment to an illusion of omnipotence. This seems to indicate the influence of Freud's 'Formulations on the two principles of mental functioning' (Freud, 1911a) where he opposes hallucination (and what he describes as 'phantasying') to reality testing. According to Petot this brought two major points in Klein's early works together: where sublimation of sexual curiosity and strengthening of the sense of reality correlates with the decline of the feeling of omnipotence (Petot, 1990).

We can see that in the beginning Klein's preoccupation was related to the issue of inhibition. She saw libido as the prime psychic mover and believed in the existence of an epistemophilic instinct rooted in libido and expressed in all the child's activities (Spillius, 1994). Aggression was seen as a component of the libidinal (sexual) drive. It was from 1926 when, through her work with young children, she recognized the importance of early aggressive impulses such as an archaic oral sadism, and from 1932, when she started to incorporate Freud's concept of the death instinct (Petot, 1990) that play activities and phantasies were seen to be attached to both life and death drives. Similarly, at this first stage she still saw anxiety arising as a consequence of repression of the Oedipus Complex. Here Klein was still following Freud and Abraham's libidinal phases theory. With the acceptance of Freud's theory of the death instinct formulated in 'Beyond the pleasure principle' (Freud, 1920a) she modified her theory of anxiety, linking it with the threat to the ego arising from the death instinct.

In this first period of development of her theories Klein saw school inhibitions evolving from the earliest play-inhibitions. She proposed that castration fear, originating sometimes from a castrating father and at other times from a castrating mother, is the common basis for these early and for all subsequent inhibitions. She thought that in order to reverse this process, given the origin of these inhibitions, there was a need for an early analysis that 'should remove the inhibitions more or less present in every child, and work at school should start on this foundation' (Klein, 1923a, p. 76).

Klein's idea of education as a prophylaxis against future neurosis differed significantly from Hug-Hellmuth's ideas, in which the curative and educational work of analysis aimed not only to free the child from his suffering but also to 'furnish him with moral and aesthetic values' (Hug-Hellmuth, 1921).

Klein came to realize that Fritz's inhibitions could not be solved only through sexual enlightenment. Fritz showed a disinclination to assimilate certain knowledge even when the information was given, mainly concerning parental intercourse and the father's role in it. Sometimes, information endlessly repeated to him met a very strong resistance. He also needed to hold on to his omnipotence of thought and to his belief that he could make things happen if he wished to. Even though sexual enlightenment had good effects, his neurotic difficulties were not sufficiently alleviated. When Klein presented her results at the Hungarian Psychoanalytical Society in 1919, Anton von Freund suggested she was dealing only with conscious phenomena, taking into account the child's conscious curiosity rather than what lay in his unconscious. Von Freund also suggested that she distinguish analytic time from other activities and that she set a fixed time for it (Petot, 1979, p. 29). Klein followed his recommendation and set a certain time apart for Fritz's analysis. Educational motives were left aside and Klein started to focus more and more on the child's anxieties and on the defences against them (Klein, 1955b, p. 123).

This first period brought some very important new developments in Klein's thinking – such as the equivalence of play, dreams and phantasy as manifestations of the child's unconscious, and a first approach in understanding the mechanism of splitting (Petot, 1979, p. 35). Fritz communicated that he was afraid of witches. He was very frightened of one of Grimm's fairy-tales where a witch offers a man poisoned food but instead of eating it, he hands it on to his horse, which dies of it. Fritz insisted that there were beautiful queens who were witches too. Klein asked him why he was afraid of something so bad coming from his mother, what had he wished about her? Fritz replied that when he had been angry he had wished that both her and his father should die and that he had thought 'dirty mamma' (Klein, 1921, p. 41). Klein understood the witch as a figure obtained by the division of the mother-imago. We can see Klein's use here of both the concept of splitting and of projection (later described in theory as projective identification; see Chapter 9).

First analysis

Klein resumed the analysis of Fritz in Berlin, when he was about seven. In her 1955 paper on the psychoanalytic play technique (1955b), Klein explains the beginning of her analytic experience with children:

> My first patient was a five-year old boy. I referred to him under the name 'Fritz' in my earliest published paper ['The development of a child', Klein, 1921]. To begin with I thought it would be sufficient to influence the mother's attitude. I suggested she should encourage the child to discuss freely with her the many unspoken questions which were obviously at the back of his mind and were impeding his intellectual development. This had a good effect but his neurotic difficulties were not sufficiently alleviated and it was soon decided that I should psycho-analyse him. ... I interpreted what I thought to be most urgent in the material the child presented to me and found my interest focusing on his anxieties and the defences

against them. ... The treatment was carried out in the child's home with his own toys. This analysis was the beginning of the psycho-analytic play technique, because from the start the child expressed his phantasies and anxieties mainly in play, and I consistently interpreted its meaning to him, with the result that additional material came up in his play. (Klein, 1955b, p. 123)

The analysis of Fritz, together with that of Felix, a 13-year-old boy who suffered from tics, was followed by the analysis of a number of children whom she saw in Berlin.

Felix experienced severe inhibitions towards school tasks as well as with social relations. The analysis of Felix enabled Klein to gain insight into the way puberty intensified the boy's difficulties. Felix had gone through a stretching of the foreskin of his penis at the age of three and the connection between this and masturbation was very strong in him. He had shared his parents' bedroom up to the age of six and had had to cope with the birth of a baby brother when he was seven. His father had threatened him into giving up masturbation. During his first years at school he had been very anxious about playing games and going to the gym, prompting threats from his father who had accused him of cowardice. The boy had overcome his anxiety by becoming an ardent footballer, but responded to his father's insistence on supervising his homework by losing interest in his schoolwork (Klein, 1925).

Klein thought castration anxiety and the boy's incessant struggle against masturbation dominated his development. Felix described his difficulties in completing a school exercise in a similar way to that in which he described his attempts at masturbation, both becoming prone to a particular rhythm: 'fast-faster-slower-and not finishing' (Klein, 1923b, p. 63). Through analysis of the boy's conscious phantasies, Klein arrived at an understanding of his unconscious phantasy of taking his mother's place in relation to the father in a passive homosexual attitude. The analysis brought a change in the content of Felix's masturbation phantasies in that their homosexual content changed from passive to active, subsequently moving to a heterosexual object choice. The boy showed a renewed interest in school subjects and overcame his anxiety at masturbating. The analysis of the tic revealed its connection with repressed masturbation wishes and the primal scene, and the tic disappeared concurrently with the appearance of heterosexual desires.

The connection that Klein made between Felix's whole emotional development and the successive transformations of his masturbatory phantasies, and the way these phantasies are seen to organize and express the boy's object relations during his development and his analysis, led Petot to propose that Klein was already working with an implicit assumption that all psychological activity and behaviour comprised the expression and realization of unconscious phantasy (Petot, 1990, p. 56; see also Chapter 2).

In 1924 Klein started analysing a number of children in Berlin: Ruth, Trude, Peter and Erna. She gained experience with these analyses, but it was the analysis of a girl aged two years and nine months, whom she called Rita, that was going to prove decisive for the development of her theories.

Rita suffered from night terrors, animal phobias, moodiness and the inability to tolerate deprivations. She was very ambivalent towards her mother, rejecting her as well as clinging to and being unable to leave her. She constantly asked her mother 'Am I good?' 'Do you love me?' Rita also showed strong obsessional features, as well as problems with eating, and a marked inhibition in play. The only thing she could do with her dolls was to wash them and change their clothes in a compulsive way (Klein, 1945, 1955b). The little girl had shared her parents' bedroom until she was nearly two, and had repeatedly witnessed sexual intercourse between her parents. The outbreak of the neurosis coincided with the birth of her little brother when she was two years old.

Klein saw Rita at the child's home. In her first session, Rita became quite anxious and said she wanted to go outside. Klein went with her to the garden and interpreted the little girl's anxiety as fear that Klein would do something to her while alone with her in the room, and she linked this to Rita's night terrors. Rita's anxiety eased, she became friendly and readily agreed to go back into the room. This case strengthened Klein's conviction of the need to interpret the child's anxieties and phantasies from the very beginning, that the:

> exploration of the unconscious is the main task of psycho-analytic procedure, and that the analysis of the transference is the means of achieving this aim. (Klein, 1955b, p. 123)

This included the interpretation of the negative transference from the beginning, whenever this was felt to be relevant.

The psychoanalytic play technique

Klein's discovery of the psychoanalytic play technique was fundamental to the development of her theories. As is often the case with scientific discoveries, the finding of new tools opened the door to important new developments. It could be compared with Freud's discovery of 'free association'. At the same time, to be able to 'discover' a new tool requires an important degree of insight and open-mindedness, as with Freud's abandonment of the 'pressure technique' in favour of 'free association'. Klein followed the children's own initiatives and was able to allow them to lead her on the path to further exploration. As Klein herself expressed it: 'if one approaches child-analysis with an open mind one will discover ways and means of probing to the deepest depths' (Klein, 1927, p. 142).

Play is the natural way a child communicates with others, as well as with himself. It enables the child to explore the external world, as well as to work through phantasies and master his anxieties. In his play the child dramatizes his conscious and unconscious phantasies. Klein concludes that the child's free play and the varied activities he displays in the consulting room are the means of expressing what the adult expresses predominantly through words, and serve the same purpose as the adult's free associations (Klein, 1955b; Segal, 1979). For Klein, child's play is serious mental work, sometimes equivalent to dreams:

> In their play children represent symbolically phantasies, wishes and experiences. Here they are employing the same language, the same archaic, phylogenetically acquired mode of expression as we are familiar with from dreams. We can only fully understand it if we approach it by the method Freud has evolved for unravelling dreams. Symbolism is only a part of it: if we want rightly to comprehend children's play in connection with their whole behaviour during the analytic hour, we must take into account not only the symbolism which often appears so clearly in their games, but also all the means of representation and the mechanisms employed in dream-work, and we must bear in mind the necessity of examining the whole nexus of phenomena. (Klein, 1926, p. 134)

Toys have a specific symbolic meaning to the child. This meaning varies according to the child's phantasies. A particular game, such as undressing a doll, can represent a multiplicity of phantasies: curiosity about the child's own genitals; masturbation phantasies; a wish to see and maybe to get inside the mother's body; an identification with the mother – the doll can represent a penis as well as a baby. It might also represent the baby that has been stolen from the mother etc. The material that children produce during the analytic hour should be thought of in conjunction with the manner in which they play, the reasons for changing from one game to another, as well as the means they choose for their representations. We should take into account that all of this is part of the transference relationship to the analyst and should therefore be seen as emerging and having meaning in that specific context. This has been mentioned by Klein and later developed by Betty Joseph in her description of transference as a 'total situation', meaning that everything of importance in the patient's psychic organization will be lived out in some way in the transference (Joseph, 1985; see also Chapter 13).

Klein was very careful not to attempt any 'wild' symbolic interpretations of children's play. She would wait for the child to give expression to the same psychic material in various forms (i.e. through the use of toys, drawings, cuttings, water etc.). When she felt she had arrived at an insight she interpreted the phenomena and linked them with the Unconscious and the analytic situation (Klein, 1927). Klein used a rather concrete part-object bodily language when making interpretations to her child-patients, assuming this was the language closest to unconscious phantasies, and so tried to reach the children at the level she felt was most appropriate to them. The formulation of interpretations has changed since these early days. There is today more of a tendency to concentrate on the immediate experience in the transference, with a greater emphasis on function (i.e. thinking, evacuating, seeing). It seems important though not to lose sight of the infantile levels of experience and phantasy that are expressed in the here and now. Spillius stresses the importance of listening to both levels of expression together (Spillius, 1994, p. 351).

In a paper presented at the British Psycho-Analytical Society on 4 May 1927, Klein discussed some of the main aspects of her views on child analysis, comparing them with Hug-Hellmuth's and Anna Freud's views on the subject. Hermine Von Hug-Hellmuth was already analysing children in Vienna by 1920, but she laid stress on the importance of the educative guidance of the analyst: 'the aim of child-analysis is character analysis – in other words, education' (Hug-Hellmuth, 1921). Klein stressed her conviction that the psychoanalyst should not exert any educative influence on the child and that a 'true analytic situation can be brought about only by analytic means' (Klein, 1927, p. 143).

The issue of the development of a transference relationship to the analyst was one of the points of disagreement between Anna Freud and Melanie Klein. Anna Freud's initial opinion was that transference in childhood is restricted to single 'transference reactions' and did not develop into a complete transference neurosis. She later modified her former opinion though she was still unconvinced that transference neurosis in children could equal the adult variety (Freud, 1966, p. 36). Klein thought that children developed a real transference to the analyst, on the basis of the child's projection on to the analyst of internal parental figures. It was those figures pertaining to the internal world, and not the real external parents, which formed the basis of transference (Segal, 1967). Klein's concept of transference included the notion of an internal object (see Chapter 8). The transference observed in the psychoanalysis of children was based on the phantasies and feelings towards introjected objects. It was therefore appropriate to make transference interpretations to a child. Klein thought that the only way to diminish the child's anxiety was to interpret the negative transference when it was felt to be operating, from the beginning, and to trace it back to the original object. She saw it as a grave error to try to ensure that the child developed a positive transference (Klein, 1927, p. 143). She did not permit child-patients any personal gratifications, in the form of either presents or caresses. From the very beginning Klein gave priority to analysing the sources of the child's anxiety.

Klein encountered in very young children a superego of a tyrannical severity apparently far in excess of anything justified by the behaviour of the real parents, and she thought that the child's immature ego could not come to terms with his superego. She thought it very important not to identify the real objects (that is, the real external parents) with those introjected by the child (Klein, 1927). This does not mean that Klein under-estimated the possibility that parents were capable of having a negative influence on their child. She frequently acknowledged parents' own neuroses and difficulties. She was also well aware that for unconscious reasons parents might hinder the work done with their child, and that anyone who analyses children had to reckon with a certain hostility and jealousy in their parents. But this was not the focus of her interpretations. Her belief was that when a child became less neurotic, he could exercise a favourable influence on the relationship with his parents.

In 1923 Klein undertook the analysis of a seven-year-old girl who had school difficulties. She was reserved, silent and rather unresponsive. During a session when she felt that she was not getting any further in the analysis, Klein picked up some of her own children's toys and brought them to the session. The child became interested and at once began to play. The girl played with two toy figures in such a way that it always ended in catastrophe. This was repeated with signs of mounting anxiety. Klein inferred, and interpreted to the child, that some sexual activity seemed to have occurred between her and a friend of hers, and that she had become very frightened of being found out, and of the teacher who was seen to be the one who would find out and punish her. This was also linked to the transference and then to the relationship to the girl's mother. The effect of this interpretation was described by Klein as striking: the child's anxiety and distrust gave way to relief, she became more friendly and less suspicious (Klein, 1955b). The regular use of toys became the means to reach the child's phantasies and anxieties.

The main principles underlying the type of toys chosen by Klein are still in place today. The chosen toys should be simple (according to Klein preferably small and easy to handle). They should enable the child to express a wide range of phantasies and experiences. Klein used little wooden men and women, cars, trains, airplanes, animals, bricks, houses, fences, paper, pencils, paints, glue, balls or marbles, plasticine and string (Klein, 1955b). Many of these basic toys are still used today in the analysis of children. There has been some modification in appropriate cases, such as the use of non-miniature dolls with children who have been sexually abused, and of toys more akin to a toddler's domestic world for very ill patients such as autistic children who have little capacity for symbolic play (Rustin, 1997).

The equipment of the room should be very simple and ideally include the possibility of playing with water. Games with water give the analyst a deep insight into the pre-genital impulses of the child, as well as offering a means of illustrating his sexual theories (Bronstein, 1997). The analyst has to be careful not to inhibit the child's aggressive phantasies but should not allow physical attacks on herself. It is therefore useful to have a room (preferably a separate room used only for child analysis), which can withstand some minor damage without disturbing the analyst's capacity to function (Joseph, 1998).

It is important for the child to be able to keep all his playthings locked in a drawer or a box that becomes part of the private relationship between analyst and patient and of the psychoanalytic transference situation. To give an example, a nine-year-old girl, whom I will call Jane, could not use any of the material she was given. She had suffered from quite a lot of neglect from her mother who was mentally ill. Jane was living with another family and even though she missed her mother she did not want to see her. In her sessions Jane regularly tore every pencil, toy and piece of paper into bits and kept all the pieces in her box. Her box ended up containing bits of paper as well as broken bits of toys. She became terrified of opening it. It seemed as if she was, in phantasy, controlling all these bits, which contained her own aggression, by leaving them inside the box. She could then have a 'good' relationship with me, having eliminated all signs of aggression. But it became clear that this splitting did not work as she felt that the box was persecuting her even when closed. At certain points she did not want to enter the room because the box was there. The box represented her internal world, full of frightening aggressive bits, as well as her ill mother whom she felt she had attacked and was attacked by.

The relationship with her internal damaged mother was felt by Jane to be beyond reparation and she felt persecuted by intense guilt that induced in her a compulsion to destroy all her toys. Understanding this, and the unconscious reasons behind it, helped her to be able to open the box and look at what she had done. By then she wasn't too frightened that I would become all 'bad', and she could see me as trying to help her meet her internal reality. Slowly, she became able to discriminate what should be thrown away from what was still intact and usable or could be repaired, as well as being able to express guilt and sadness for having destroyed some good valuable toys. She finally managed to play with what was left and created a number of drawings and paintings that she left inside her box and was very pleased to find again in her next session.

The psychoanalytic play technique is the central tool in the analysis and psychotherapy of children. Klein's discoveries promoted the development of this field of knowledge and the possibility that children could have access to psychotherapeutic help from early infancy. Bion's understanding of the maternal role of containment of anxiety as fundamental to the development in the baby of the capacity to think was one among many important contributions to this field by Klein's followers (Bion, 1962a; see also Chapter 12).

Understanding the uncertainty, confusion and anxiety experienced by the mother of a newborn baby was another area of study promoted by Klein's theories. Harris considered that the analyst's anxiety when exposed to uncertainty resembled the new mother's anxiety when bombarded by the emotional state of the infant:

> The essential intimacy and nakedness of the analyst–patient relationship, if an analytic process is taking place ... is probably more analogous to the mother–baby relationship than to any other. (Harris, 1976, p. 226)

These ideas contributed to the development and incorporation of 'infant observation' as a necessary requirement in the training of child psychotherapists and psychoanalysts in England.

Klein's first theories

Melanie Klein's first psychoanalytical ideas were based on Freud's first theory of anxiety, that is, that discharge in the form of anxiety is the consequence of repression of libido. She came to the conclusion that every time anxiety was resolved the analysis took a big step forward, and that the degree of success in removing inhibitions was in direct proportion to the clarity with which anxiety manifested itself (Klein, 1923b). This conceptualization changed with the understanding of early sadism in the infant.

From the analysis of Rita, Klein came to some theoretical conclusions which introduced practical and technical changes in her treatment of children. On the practical side, Klein realized that psychoanalysis could not be carried out in the child's home, however small the child was. She found that the home atmosphere could be hostile to the analyst and that the transference situation could not be maintained unless the patient felt that the analysis was something separate from the ordinary home life:

> For only under such conditions can he overcome his resistances against experiencing and expressing thoughts, feelings, and desires, which are incompatible with convention, and in the case of children, felt to be in contrast to much of what they have been taught. (Klein, 1955b, p. 125)

On the theoretical side, she recognized the early onset of anxiety situations which she linked to aggressive impulses rather than to repression of libido, thus following Freud's second theory of anxiety.

From the very beginning of her work Klein placed great importance on the child's interest in and curiosity toward his mother's body, and on the effects that repression of these wishes have on the child. For example, she thought that the basis of a child's inhibition of the sense of orientation arose from the need to repress his interest in his mother's womb and its contents, such as the desire to penetrate the mother's body and to investigate it inside. Repression of these wishes could lead to inhibitions of this faculty:

> Abraham pointed out that the interest in orientation in relation to the body of the mother is preceded at a very early stage by the interest in orientation in relation to the subject's own body. This is certainly true, but this early orientation seems to share the fate of repression only when the interest in orientation in reference to the mother's body is repressed, of course because of the incestuous wishes bound up with that interest; for in the unconscious the longed-for return to the womb and exploration of it takes place by way of coitus. (Klein, 1923b, p. 98)

By 1928 Klein had described an early connection between the epistemophilic instinct and sadism which was activated by the rise of Oedipal tendencies and which 'at first mainly concerns itself with the mother's body, which is assumed to be the scene of all sexual processes and developments' (Klein, 1928, p. 188). The desire to take possession of the mother's body ushered in a phase of development in both sexes which she named the 'femininity phase'. In this first period of the development of her theories Klein followed Abraham's ideas on the oral cannibalistic stage of development. She described a phase that began with the emergence of oral-sadistic instincts and ended with the decline of the earlier anal stage in which she thought sadism was at its height (Klein, 1933).

Rita's early sadism manifested itself in unconscious phantasies of attacking her mother's body, wishing to rob and kill her. This evoked in her the fear of being abandoned by a 'good' mother and terror of a 'bad' mother destroying her body and its contents, and taking the children out of it (Klein, 1932, pp. 29, 31). Klein postulated a theory of an archaic Oedipus Complex which differed from Freud's conceptualization of the Oedipus Complex, not only in terms of timing, but also in its characteristics (Klein, 1926, p. 129). Klein believed that the Oedipus Complex had a powerful influence at an early age, with Oedipal desires coming to the fore at the end of the first year, and that the little girl's choice of father as a love-object ensued after weaning. She thought at this point that weaning, plus the training in cleanliness, made the girl turn to her father whose caresses were construed by the little girl as seduction. As early as 1923 Klein had the image of 'maternal castration', as in the case of Fritz (Klein, 1923a, p. 64). She actually thought that both sexes turned away from the mother's frustrating breast to the father's penis. Klein's first theory of the Oedipus Complex was later modified with the development of her theory of the depressive position (see Chapter 6).

The aggression felt towards the mother was felt to endanger the loved mother and brought anxiety and guilt. Klein found for example that many of Rita's symptoms were due to a strong sense of guilt (Klein, 1945). Awareness of very early feelings of guilt and of early reparation mechanisms led her to think of an early super-ego. This primitive super-ego was a much earlier structure than it had been for Freud, and was not necessarily the heir of the Oedipus Complex, as early introjections of pre-genital forms entered into its development.

This first period in the development of her psychoanalytic theories formed the basis of Klein's future explorations. Even though many of her initial propositions were later modified, they provided the bedrock from which she could move forward, developing and expanding her theories of the mind.

CHAPTER 2

Freud and Klein on the concept of phantasy

ELIZABETH BOTT SPILLIUS

One of Freud's earliest discoveries was that in the Unconscious, memories and phantasies are not distinguished – hence his abandonment of his earliest theory of neurosis, the 'seduction' or 'affect trauma' theory. From that time onwards phantasies have been of central interest. In this chapter I will discuss the ideas of Freud and Klein on this most interesting and complex concept; then I will discuss my own use of it in two psychoanalytic sessions.

Considering its importance, it is perhaps surprising that Freud did not devote even a paper to the concept of phantasy, let alone a book. His ideas on it are scattered about in the first twenty years of his psychoanalytic writings. His most explicit theoretical statements about it are to be found in his paper 'Formulations on the two principles of mental functioning' in 1911 and in Lecture 23 of the *Introductory Lectures in Psycho-Analysis* (1916). In her work with children Klein gradually developed a rather different view from that of Freud. Klein's view was explicitly stated by Susan Isaacs (1948) and was the central theoretical issue of the Controversial Discussions in the British Psycho-Analytical Society in 1943 (King and Steiner, 1991). The various views on phantasy voiced at the Discussions are clearly described and discussed by Anne Hayman (1989).

One of the difficulties in expounding the differences between Freud's and Klein's views on phantasy is that Freud uses the term rather differently in different places. In 'Formulations on the two principles of mental functioning', which is the place where he comes closest to making a formal definition, he speaks of phantasy as a wish-fulfilling activity which can arise when an instinctual wish is frustrated. Phantasies derive ultimately from unconscious impulses, the basic instincts of sex and aggression. I shall call this Freud's 'central usage'. (It is well expounded by Sandler and Nagera, 1963.)

17

In understanding Freud's central usage it is important to remember that his idea of phantasy, like his work on dreams, is closely bound up with the development of his topographical model of the mind (see Chapter 7 of *The Interpretation of Dreams*, 1900, SE 5; his papers 'Repression', 1915d; and 'The unconscious', 1915e; Sandler *et al.*, 1997). In the topographical model of the mind, conceptualized as the System Unconscious, the System Preconscious, and the System Conscious, there is a double focus, first on the attributes of consciousness and unconsciousness, and secondly on primary and secondary process. The 'secondary process' Freud defined as the rational thinking of ordinary logic; the 'primary process' he thought of as a much more peculiar system of logic, characteristic of the System Unconscious, in which opposites are equated, there is no sense of time, no negation, no conflict.

Although Freud thought that some unconscious phantasies might be 'unconscious all along', he thought that most phantasies originated as conscious or preconscious daydreams and might subsequently be repressed. As he puts it in 'Hysterical phantasies and their relation to bisexuality' (1908), the unconscious phantasies of hysterics 'have either been unconscious all along and have been formed in the unconscious; or – as is more often the case – they were once conscious phantasies, day-dreams, and have since been purposely forgotten and have become unconscious through 'repression' (1908, p. 161). In Freud's view the basic motive force for making phantasies is an unconscious wish that is blocked from fulfilment, and the phantasy is a disguised expression and partial fulfilment of this unconscious wish. If phantasies are formed in the System Conscious or if they are allowed into it, that is, if they are daydreams, they are known not to be true. If they are formed in the System Preconscious or if they are repressed into it, they will be descriptively unconscious but formed according to the everyday logic of the secondary process. If phantasies are further repressed into the System Unconscious, they become subject to the peculiar logic of the primary process; they 'proliferate in the dark', as Freud put it, and from their position in the System Unconscious they may become indistinguishable from memories and may also find their way into dreams, symptoms, symptomatic acts, further preconscious and conscious phantasies, and other drive derivatives.

Freud's 'central usage, with its emphasis on phantasies being formed according to the logical thinking of the secondary process, is the usage that was adopted by Anna Freud, by the Viennese analysts during the Controversial Discussions, and by several British analysts, notably Marjorie Brierley (King and Steiner, 1991). This is the usage that has been adopted by ego psychologists, the Contemporary Freudian group of analysts in Britain, and also by many independent analysts (see Hayman, 1989).

In Freud's view, although there *are* phantasies in the System Unconscious, the basic unit of the System Unconscious is not phantasy but the unconscious instinctual wish. The making of dreams and the making of phantasies are parallel processes; one might speak of 'phantasy work' as comparable to the 'dream work'; both involve transformation of primary unconscious content into a disguised form. For Klein, on the contrary, unconscious phantasies *are* the primary unconscious content, and dreams are a transformation of it. For Freud, the prime mover, so to speak, is the unconscious wish; dreams and phantasies are both disguised derivatives of it. For Klein the prime mover is unconscious phantasy.

I think that Freud and Klein emphasized contrasting aspects of the everyday usage of the word 'phantasy'. The word contains an inherent contradiction both in English and I believe also in German. It has a connotation of the imagination and creativity that underlie all thought and feeling, but it also has a connotation of make believe, a daydream, something that is untrue by the standards of material reality (see Rycroft, 1968; Laplanche and Pontalis, 1973; Steiner, 1988; Britton, 1995). Freud's central usage emphasizes the fictitious, wish-fulfilling aspect of the everyday usage whereas Klein's usage tends to focus on the imaginative aspect.

But this relatively clear-cut contrast between Freud and Klein is complicated by the fact that Freud's 'central usage' is not by any means his only usage. Further, he moves easily from one implied definition to another without being finicky about his formulations. In some of his early work he seems at times almost to equate unconscious phantasy with unconscious wish (1900, p. 574); at others he speaks of phantasies largely as conscious or preconscious daydreams (1900, pp. 491–8). In his clinical work he deduces phantasies of quite surprising content, phantasies of which the patient was presumably unaware. He assumes, for example, that the Wolf Man when he was one and a half years old had a phantasy of being inside his mother's womb so as to intercept his father's penis (1920b, pp. 101–3). It is not clear whether Freud thought the Wolf Man was consciously aware of this phantasy at the time and repressed it later, or whether it never became conscious at all. Freud deduces similarly striking phantasies in the case of Dora (1905a), though he does not discuss their precise topographical status. Some of Dora's phantasies were presumably conscious, such as her phantasy of revenge on her father. Some were probably at least descriptively unconscious, such as her phantasy of fellatio, of the female genital (the 'nymphs' in the 'thick wood', that is, the labia minora in the pubic hair), her phantasy of defloration, of bearing Herr K's child, and her homosexual love for Frau K.

It seems likely that Freud always tacitly assumed that at least some phantasies may originate directly in the System Unconscious without being originally preconscious or conscious derivatives of unconscious wishes. Indeed in 1916 he speaks of 'primal phantasies' which he thinks are inherited; these are the phantasies of the primal scene, of castration, of seduction by an adult. He does not mean, he makes clear, that parental intercourse is never seen, that threats of castration do not occur, or that seduction does not happen in reality. But he thinks that these phantasies will occur even if external reality does not support them because they were once, to quote him, 'real occurrences in the primeval times of the human family, and that children in their phantasies are simply filling in the gaps in individual truth with prehistoric truth' (Lecture 23 of the *Introductory Lectures*, 1916, p. 371). Most of Freud's followers have not adopted this view, thinking of it as too Lamarckian. But with some alteration I think it is not far away from Klein's notion of inherent knowledge of bodily organs or from Bion's idea of 'preconceptions' waiting to mate with experience to form conceptions (see Chapter 12).

In summary, Freud is not punctilious in his definition of phantasy. He uses the term in several senses and, as Laplanche and Pontalis point out, he is more concerned with the transformation of one sort of phantasy into one another than with any static definition (Laplanche and Pontalis, 1973, pp. 314-19). What I have called his 'central usage', however, is that one that has been adopted by most of his immediate followers.

What, then, is Klein's view of unconscious phantasy and why did it arouse so much controversy?

Basically Klein focuses on the 'unconscious all along' aspect of phantasy. She regards phantasy as a basic mental activity present in rudimentary form from birth onwards and essential for mental growth, though it can also be used defensively. Klein developed this view of phantasy through her work with children, especially through discovering that children accompanied all their activities by a constant stream of phantasy even when they were not being frustrated by external reality. As for example Fritz and the letters of the alphabet, one of many examples:

> For in his phantasies the lines in his exercise book were roads, the book itself was the whole world and the letters rode into it on motor bicycles, i.e. on the pen. Again, the pen was a boat and the exercise book a lake. ... In general he regarded the small letters as the children of the capital letters. The capital S he looked upon as the emperor of the long German s's; it had two hooks at the end of it to distinguish it from the empress, the terminal s, which had only one hook. (Klein, 1923a, p. 100)

Klein developed her idea of phantasy gradually from 1919 onwards, stressing particularly the damaging effect of inhibition of phantasy in the development of the child, the ubiquity of phantasies about the mother's body and its contents, the variety of phantasies about the primal scene and the Oedipus Complex, the intensity of both aggressive and loving phantasies, the combination of several phantasies to form what she called the depressive position – the paranoid-schizoid position was to come later, in 1946 – the development of phantasies of internal objects, and, of course, the expression of all these phantasies in the play of children and the thinking and behaviour of adults. Essentially I think that Klein viewed unconscious phantasy as synonymous with unconscious thought, and that she perhaps used the term 'phantasy' rather than 'thought' because the thoughts of her child patients were more imaginative and less rational than ordinary adult thought is supposed to be. Further, Klein thought that it was possible to deduce the phantasies of infants from her analyses of small children, assuming that she was discovering the infant in the child much as Freud had discovered the child in the adult (Britton, 1995).

So important was the concept of phantasy in Klein's thinking that the British Society made it the central scientific topic of the Controversial Discussions of the 1940s (King and Steiner, 1991), the aim of the discussions being to see whether Klein's ideas were to be regarded as heresy or development. It was Susan Isaacs, however, who gave the definitive paper, 'The nature and function of phantasy' (1948). In it Isaacs stressed the link between Klein's concept of phantasy and Freud's concept of drive. She defined phantasy as 'the primary content of unconscious mental processes', 'the mental corollary, the psychic representative, of instinct' (Isaacs, 1948). Phantasies are the equivalent of what Freud meant by the 'instinctual representative' or the 'psychic representative of an instinctual drive'.

Isaacs, like Klein, particularly emphasizes the idea that everyone has a continual stream of unconscious phantasy, and, further, that abnormality or normality rest not on the presence or absence of unconscious phantasy but on how it is expressed, modified, and related to external reality. She distinguishes between conscious and unconscious phantasy and suggests the 'ph' spelling to distinguish the latter. (Nowadays most British analysts use the 'ph' spelling for all phantasies, I believe because it is sometimes difficult to be sure whether phantasies are conscious or unconscious.)

Isaacs' and Klein's definition of phantasy is thus much wider than Freud's central usage. In the Kleinian view, unconscious phantasy is the mainspring, the original and essential content of the unconscious mind. It includes very early forms of infantile thought, but it also includes other forms that emerge later on in development. Freud's central usage, the wish-fulfilling definition of phantasy, is a specific and more limited form, a particular type of phantasy within Klein's more inclusive definition. In the Controversial Discussions Klein and Isaacs did not stress this relation between their all-inclusive definition and the wish-fulfilling definition of phantasy as a particular type within it. Certainly the argument in the Discussions was made more difficult by the fact that each faction was using the same word for a different concept; much of the time the two factions talked past each other. Sometimes the Viennese seemed to assume that Klein's definition of phantasy was the same as their own, so that they could not understand how Klein could possibly say that phantasies occurred in very early infantile life, since this would have meant that very small infants were capable of secondary process thinking. At other times Glover and Anna Freud specifically criticized Klein for broadening the concept of phantasy so much that it included everything and hence had become meaningless. Ronald Britton has suggested that Isaacs probably did not fully clarify the difference in definitions because she did not want to emphasize Klein's difference from Freud, for Klein and her colleagues were worried that Glover might succeed in banishing them from the Society on the grounds that they differed from Freud and were therefore not 'legitimate' (Britton, 1998b).

Freud is not very specific in making conjectures about the nature of early infantile thought. Klein called such thought phantasy and assumed that it was closely linked to bodily experience. She assumes that phantasizing starts very early, in some primitive form 'from the beginning' as she was fond of saying. She did not bother much about Freud's distinction between the System Unconscious and the System Preconscious, between primary and secondary process thinking (see Chapter 11). Klein and Isaacs assumed that phantasies could be formed according to primary process thinking – indeed that primary and secondary process thinking were very much intertwined.

Isaacs assumes that the earliest phantasies are experienced mainly as visceral sensations and urges, the other senses of touch, smell, sound, taste, and sight being added later and gradually. Such unconscious phantasies can perhaps be regarded as similar to the 'thing presentations' that Freud describes in 'The Unconscious' (1915e). Isaacs makes much use of the principle of genetic continuity to link these very early phantasies with the more structured verbal phantasies of the older child and the adult. She assumes that what is experienced is a sensation and an impulse, together with a feeling of something happening that is involved with the sensation and may have an effect on it; looked at from the perspective of an outside observer, the 'something' is some aspect of external reality. From the perspective of the infant, things are assumed to be inside him. Hinshelwood describes it as follows:

> An unconscious phantasy is a belief in the activity of concretely felt 'internal' objects. This is a difficult concept to grasp. A somatic sensation tugs along with it a mental experience that is interpreted as a relationship with an object that wishes to cause that sensation, and is loved or hated by the subject according to whether the object is well-meaning or has evil intentions (i.e. a pleasant or unpleasant

sensation). Thus an unpleasant sensation is mentally represented as a relationship with a 'bad' object that intends to hurt and damage the subject ... Conversely, when he is fed, the infant's experience is of an object, which *we* can identify as mother, or her milk, but which *the infant* identifies as an object in his tummy benevolently motivated to cause pleasant sensations there. (Hinshelwood, 1989, pp. 34-5; emphasis in original)

Slowly through introjection and projection a complex phantasy world of self and internal objects is built up, some of it conscious, but reaching to the unconscious depths. This notion of internal objects and the internal world was and has continued to be central in Kleinian thought (see Chapter 8). This internal world is imaginary by the standards of material reality, but possesses what Freud calls 'psychic' reality, that is, to the individual concerned it feels real at some level, conscious or unconscious, and it is also real in the sense that it affects his behaviour. It is noteworthy too that in the unconscious aspects of the internal world Klein and Isaacs think of phantasies as combining both ideas and feeling, another difference from Freud, who spoke of the system Unconscious as the realm of ideas and memory traces and was never entirely resolved about the status of unconscious feelings.

Early phantasies are omnipotent: 'I want it, I've got it'; 'I don't want it, it's gone!' They are stated by Isaacs to have many attributes Freud thought to be characteristic of the primary process – no coordination of impulses, no sense of time, no contradiction, no negation. But Klein also thought of unconscious impulses and phantasies being in conflict with each other in the Unconscious; unconscious conflict between love and hate, between a good self and a bad self, between a good mother and a bad mother were conceptions she found appropriate and useful, though in Freud's topographical conceptualization wishes (and wishful phantasies) in the System Unconscious are in conflict not directly with each other but indirectly through their contact with the regulating ego.

Klein and Isaacs assume that the expression of unconscious phantasy in words comes very much later than their original sensory formulation. Indeed, some unconscious phantasies about infantile experience are never formally articulated in words, though words may be the means unconsciously used to communicate them by evoking them in an external person. To give an example: in a stormy session a young woman abused me in a most persecuting manner for being profoundly boring. This was shortly before a holiday break which she was extending by leaving early. She was consciously aware of having a long-standing grudge against her parents for leaving her when she was very young, but what she was not aware of was that she (and probably her parents as well) had a profound sense of unworthiness and inadequacy over their leaving. She assumed that if she had been loveable and interesting her parents would not have left her. In this session she became the parents leaving me as the boring, stupid, miserable child, and her anger both expressed and disguised the guilt and self-justification that she unconsciously assumed her parents had felt, that she unconsciously thought I was feeling about my holiday, and that she was feeling about leaving me first. At this point in her analysis she could not talk about or even know about these feelings; she could express them only by enacting the experience and its associated phantasies. My task as analyst was to realize that my emotions were to some extent her emotions, and to find words for the phantasies the emotions embodied.

Klein and Isaacs assume that phantasies affect the perception of external reality, but, equally, that external reality affects phantasies, that there is a continual interplay between them. This assumption, namely, that actual external events are interpreted and understood, experienced in other words, in terms of pre-existing phantasies and that phantasies may be modified to take experience of events into account, is a basic premise in Kleinian thought. The first part of this assumption caused considerable argument during the Controversial Discussions and subsequently as well, for many analysts disputed Klein's assertion that an infant or child could have, say, attacking and destructive phantasies without having been destructively attacked. In the Kleinian view such phantasies of attack may conceivably be a realization of a hereditary disposition, though they may also arise from earlier experiences of bodily sensations of discomfort, as described above in the quotation from Hinshelwood. The argument about which is primary, pre-existing phantasies or external events is an expression of a more general and in my opinion unproductive psychoanalytic argument about the relative priority of heredity and environment – unproductive because psychoanalytic evidence for deciding the issue in particular cases is usually not available.

Phantasies are now viewed by Kleinians as crucially important in the development of logical thought, as they are used as hypotheses to be confirmed or disproved by experiences of external reality, an idea explicitly added to the Kleinian conception of phantasy by Hanna Segal (1964), (see also Segal, 1997b). External reality thus often operates not only as a stimulus or cause of phantasies but as a confirmation or disproof of them. One does not have to see a breast being cut to pieces to have a phantasy of it, but for one's mother's breast to ooze blood and pus is likely to be felt as an alarming confirmation of a phantasy of attack, or a disturbing disproof of a phantasy of a loving and well-cared-for breast able to stand up to attack. The testing of phantasies against reality does not mean that earlier more omnipotent phantasies are necessarily abandoned; they remain but are added to by more sophisticated versions in keeping with experiences of external reality. And often the more sophisticated versions are used to deny the psychic reality of the cruder and perhaps earlier phantasies (Britton, 1995).

Klein and Isaacs assume that phantasies are not used solely to express unconscious impulses and wishes. Mechanisms of defence too are expressed through phantasy. Projection, introjection, splitting, idealization, denial, repression are abstract terms that describe general psychic processes, but a given individual's use of them is expressed through a particular phantasy.

Phantasies expressing particular impulses and defences do not operate in isolation. Gradually they are built up into a complex system which is the individual's own unique way of being, of relating to the world, of maintaining his balance. The concept of phantasy is thus central to the idea of the organization of the personality as a whole.

It is hardly surprising that in the Controversial Discussions of the 1940s Anna Freud, Glover and their associates were not convinced by Isaacs' arguments nor she by theirs. As I have said, they meant such different things by the same term, phantasy, that they were talking past each other. I think it is worth asking, however, what is the effect on our clinical approach of these differing conceptions of phantasy. The effects should not be exaggerated. All analysts, regardless of school of thought, and regardless of their definition of the concept of phantasy, use the idea of unconscious thoughts and feelings. In Kleinian analysis such thoughts and feelings are called unconscious phantasy; in classical analysis they are called drive derivatives, and the term phantasy is used only for one particular form of drive derivative. But the conception of unconscious thoughts and feelings is of crucial importance to all analysts.

In the case of classical analysis, though I cannot speak with certainty, it seems to me that the concept of phantasy is used relatively rarely and more usually in its conscious than its unconscious form; further, only a few papers have been written about it, and they are mainly clarifications of Freud's views and further examinations of them in terms of the structural model (see Beres, 1962; Sandler and Nagera, 1963; Arlow, 1969a, 1969b; Sandler and Sandler, 1986, though in this paper the Sandlers go beyond Freud's formulations to link the concept of unconscious phantasy with their later formulations of the past and present unconscious). As I have described above, Freud himself made daring leaps in deducing the content of phantasies. Nowadays such imaginative interpretation of phantasies and dreams is more rare; clinical work is more focused on ego defences. There is perhaps an exception in the case of J. and A.M. Sandler, with their reintroduction of the topographical model and their use of the term 'fantasy' instead of 'impulse' because 'in all these impulses relations between self and object representations are involved and ... the defensive transformations that occur in the present unconscious involve to a substantial degree, modifications of fantasy interaction between self and object' (Sandler and Sandler, 1984, 373n; see also Sandler and Sandler, 1983, 1986 and 1987).

Klein's discoveries about the phantasies of small children led her to be very aware of their intense bodily concreteness, their concern with birth, death, the primal scene, babies, faeces, urine, murderous hatred and equally violent love. Her descriptions of phantasies are as graphic and surprising as those of Freud. For example:

> One day while Ruth was once again devoting her attention exclusively to her sister, she drew a picture of a tumbler with some small round balls inside and a kind of lid on top. I asked her what the lid was for, but she would not answer me. On her sister repeating the question, she said it was 'to prevent the balls from rolling out'. Before this, she had gone through her sister's bag and then shut it tightly 'so that nothing should fall out of it'. She had done the same with the purse inside the bag so as to keep the coins safely shut up ... I now made a venture and told Ruth that the balls in the tumbler, the coins in the purse and the contents of the bag all meant children in her Mummy's inside, and that she wanted to keep them safely shut up so as not to have any more brothers and sisters. The effect of my interpretation was astonishing. For the first time Ruth turned her attention to me and began to play in a different, less constrained way. (Klein, 1932, pp. 26-7)

Or again:

> As I was putting a wet sponge beside one of them [a doll] as she had done, she burst out crying again and screamed, 'No, she mustn't have the big sponge, that's not for children, that's for grown ups!' I may remark that in her two previous sessions she had brought up a lot of material concerning her envy of her mother. I now interpreted this material in connection with her protest against the big sponge which represented her father's penis. I showed her in every detail how she envied and hated her mother because the latter had incorporated her father's penis during coitus, and how she wanted to steal his penis and the children out of her mother's inside and kill her mother. I explained to her that this was why she was frightened and believed that she had killed her mother or would be deserted by her. ... Gradually she sat up and watched the course of the play with growing interest and even began to take an active part in it herself. ... [When] the nurse came ... she was surprised to find her happy and cheerful and to see her say goodbye to me in a friendly and even affectionate way. (Klein, 1932, p. 28)

Nowadays, like our classical colleagues, many Kleinian analysts have become more cautious about interpreting phantasies so boldly and so concretely (I have discussed this in Spillius, 1988b, pp. 8-9). In spite of this change, I think that emphasis on the unconscious and on adult forms of living out infantile experiences and phantasies has remained characteristic of Kleinian analysis. Like Klein herself, her present-day followers take it for granted that in thinking, in dreaming, in creativity, in all experiencing, there is a constant and often uncomfortable mixture of logic and illogic. Further, unconscious phantasy is the mainspring of both creativity and destructiveness. It gives meaning to the external world and richness to the internal world. If there has been a change in the analysis of phantasies, it is perhaps that there is an increasing tendency to see how they are lived out in the analytic session as well as how they are expressed in symbolic content.

Considering that Kleinians regard unconscious phantasy as such an important concept, it is perhaps surprising that little has been written about it since Isaacs, even less than in the case of classical analysts (but see Segal, 1964, 1997b; Joseph, 1981; Hinshelwood, 1989; Britton, 1995). I think little has been written because the concept is now taken for granted. Much of the work on the development of thinking, for example, relies on Klein's theory of phantasy and changes in the content and functions of phantasy in the movement from the paranoid schizoid to the depressive position. Similarly much of the work on psychic equilibrium and pathological organizations uses the concept of phantasy. In fact I find it difficult to illustrate the way I use the concept clinically because it is so ubiquitous that it comes into everything. That, of course, was one of the objections that Glover, Anna Freud, and others made to Klein's usage: all mental functions were encapsulated into this one concept.

But having said that, let me describe some clinical material which illustrates a phantasy that was of central importance in the life of one of my patients; in this session it was expressed not only in dreams but also in the relationship between patient and analyst.

Mr H suffered from what Klein calls persecutory depression (Klein, 1957; Riesenberg-Malcolm, 1981). He reproached himself endlessly for being useless, a failure, damaging to everyone. In spite of his self-reproaches, however, he was not really curious about the harm he was actually doing and might have done in the past, and he seemed more interested in berating himself than in putting the damage right. The phantasies underlying his destructiveness and self-destructiveness emerged in these two sessions partly in dreams and partly through our mutual acting out in the session.

Tuesday's session
He woke very anxious having had a *dream*.

> There was an open flat space covered about two inches deep in some sort of white stuff. He doesn't know what it was - chalk? cheese? breadcrumbs? He was condemned to eat this stuff forever. Other people didn't seem to be under the same pressure.

He had no ideas about the dream, was too anxious even to tackle it. He was very stuck, hopeless, despairing. He was failing me, failing his wife, failing himself, and it was all his fault. I made several interpretations to the effect that he wanted me to feel what it was like to be helpless - I couldn't help him even to think why he was so anxious and frantic, just as he hadn't been able to help his frantic, anxious mother.

Wednesday

He had lost his cheque card and then forgot he had lost it. It was like his homework when he was a child – he used to forget to do it and then forgot he had forgotten it. There was always a vague area of persecution. (Pause) 'Why didn't my mother see to it that I did it?'

I said he was becoming curious about his forgetting and mine. He expected me, like himself and his mother, to go along with the way he loses all knowledge of what he has done and then even forgets he has forgotten. He is always guilty, but has forgotten his crime, and, indeed, doesn't even know if there was a crime.

'I think you're right,' he said. (For the first time in these two sessions there was interest in his voice.) 'I didn't want to let go,' he went on, 'I wanted to preserve the persecution. It would have been infinitely simpler to have done the homework.'

I agreed with this and added that perhaps he expected me to get tangled up in forgetting and ignoring whatever the homework might be now.

His reply to that was that he had had another *dream*.

> There was a plaque. It was my job to discover what it was. It took hours to work it out. Once I had done so, I could forget it.

He paused, then said he thought it had something to do with the area covered with crumbs in the dream of yesterday, but said he couldn't get much further.

I drew his attention to the contrast between the two dreams. In the crumbs dream he has to eat the stuff forever; in the plaque dream he has to discover what it was and then he could leave it. I said I thought perhaps both represented his analysis, about which he had such mixed feelings. Perhaps the crumbs were a way of saying that was all he got from me ...

'No!' he suddenly said. 'They weren't crumbs. It was bread, I can see it now. It was as if it had been gouged out, torn apart.'

After a pause I drew his attention to the violence of that image, as if he couldn't bear what he had done so that he made it bland and flat.

'And white!' he added, 'Very white. You're right, it's a massacre, it's white so as not to be bloody.' Pause. In this pause I was remembering material that was well-known to both of us, namely, that when he was a baby his mother had had a breast abscess so that her breast had bled when she fed him. Meanwhile Mr H went on to a new and different thought. 'I don't know why I should think of that baby who drowned,' he said. (This was a case reported in the newspaper of a baby drowning; the mother tried to rescue the baby, jumped in after him, and drowned as well.)

I said that death by drowning was the revenge he expected to be taken on him for having made so violent an attack. I thought it was an idea he had of getting inside me, inside my breast as he perhaps once felt he had got inside his mother's, tearing it apart, gouging it out, so that when it tried to feed him it would drown him in blood as well as milk. And I would drown with him because I could not feed him or save him, and this painful situation would be endlessly perpetuated.

'Christ,' he said. 'And all this is going on without a person knowing anything about it.'

It is very difficult to describe what he conveyed by the way he said this. On the one hand he seemed to be laughing at me, as if saying 'What utter nonsense my analyst talks!' On the other hand he seemed to be saying that what I had said was absolutely right, and it horrified him to think of the things he was feeling and thinking without his being aware of them. It was an odd combination of triumph and compliance. I was not quick enough to get hold of this contradiction at the time. Instead I said: 'A "person" is an odd way of putting it. Clearly you mean yourself, but I think you also mean me and your mother. I think you feel I ought to know just as your mother should have known how dreadful you felt about what was happening when you were a baby and later about your homework, and now I should realise how hopeless you feel.'

He said: 'So my punishment is to have to eat the stuff forever and ever.'

By this time I think I had lost him. He had had a moment of truth earlier in the session, but now he was slipping back into his usual melancholic rumination in which he was bad and I could not help him. If I were doing this session again, I think that is what I would say. But at the time I was optimistically trying to save him, just like the mother who tried to save her baby by jumping in after him.

In fact what I said was that I thought he had a theory that he was saving his mother and saving me by punishing himself forever. But actually what seemed gradually to be becoming clearer was that punishing himself was a way of not knowing about his own destructiveness and neglect. I said I thought his plaque dream seemed to be saying that if he could find out what it was, which I thought meant whatever he'd really done and whatever I'd really done and his mother had really done, then he could be allowed to forget. That was the end of the session.

As I have indicated, I think Mr H had an unconscious phantasy of a crime that he could not face and know and that could not be forgotten unless it was known. In the first dream it was expressed as white stuff he had to eat forever; in the second he could be allowed to forget something if he could discover what it was. His phantasy of a bloodthirsty attack disguised as bland white stuff was thus expressed in the visual symbols of the dreams, further clarified by his associations. But my patient's phantasy of attack was also unconsciously lived out in the session, and in a more subtle form than his expression of it in the dreams. It began with his realization that the bread-crumbs were white so as not to be bloody. I think he knew, given the work we had done in the past, that I would be likely to interpret this as his attack on his mother's breast and on me. Then came his sudden switch to the image of the mother jumping in after the baby and drowning too. I failed to realize at the time that I was about to jump in after my patient by making a prema-ture and overly symbolic interpretation about his attack on the breast. To this he responded by his peculiar mixture of triumph and compliance and then by relapsing into his familiar masochistic defence of punishing himself (and me, and his parents) forever.

An additional element in this interaction, which was repeated in many other sessions, was that Mr H was behaving towards me as he felt his mother had behaved towards him. She was (and is, by his account) self-centred, extremely anxious, and constantly makes my patient feel that there is nothing he can do to help her, which of course makes him angry as well as guilty. My patient punishes himself endlessly for this anger and his phantasies of attack on her, but the exquisite irony of his self-punishment is that it is based on an identification with his mother. He is as neglectful and self-indulgent as she is; he fails to thrive in his life and his work, is a constant source of worry to his parents, and thus punishes them even more than himself. And this, as you may imagine, is what he attempts to live out in his analysis over and over again.

Conclusion

In summary, I think Freud's idea is that the prime mover of psychic life is the unconscious wish, not phantasy. The 'work' of making phantasies and the 'work' of making dreams are parallel processes in which forbidden uncon-scious wishes achieve disguised expression and partial fulfilment. For Freud himself, especially in his central usage, and even more for his immediate followers, phantasies are conceived as imagined fulfilments of frustrated wishes. Whether they originate in the System Conscious or the System Preconscious, they are an activity of the ego and are formed according to the principles of the secondary process. That is not the whole story, however, because phantasies may get repressed into the System Unconscious where they become associated with the instinctual wishes, become subject to the laws of the primary process, and may find their way into dreams and many other derivatives. And there are the primal, phylogenetic phantasies, also capable of being directly incorporated into dreams.

For Klein unconscious phantasies play the part that Freud assigned to the unconscious wish. They underlie dreams rather than being parallel to them – a much more inclusive definition of phantasy than Freud's. The earliest and most deeply unconscious phantasies are bodily, and only gradually, with maturation and developing experience through introjection and projection do some of them come to take a verbal form. Freud's central usage, the wish-fulfilling definition of phantasy, is a particular type of phantasy within Klein's more inclusive definition. In Klein's usage, unconscious phantasies underlie not only dreams but all thought and activity, both creative and destructive, including the expression of internal object relations in the analytic situation.

* I am grateful to several colleagues for discussion and help in writing this paper, especially Dr H. Segal, Dr R. Steiner and Dr R. Britton.

CHAPTER 3

The paranoid-schizoid position

PRISCILLA ROTH

Terror enlarges the object; as does love. (William Carlos Williams)

Beginning in 1935, with her paper 'A contribution to the psychogenesis of manic-depressive states', and continuing through the rest of her life, Melanie Klein progressively explored and outlined what she described as two different 'positions' : *the paranoid-schizoid position*, first described in 1946, in 'Notes on some schizoid mechanisms'; and *the depressive position*, first described in 1935 and 1940.

Klein was attempting to understand and describe the earliest mental development in the infant, and, at the same time, the roots of particular descriptively distinct mental states in older children and in adults. She began with the notion that the newborn infant has certain inborn characteristics which will colour and partly determine the way he responds to and relates to his new world. And then, from her experience analysing young children and adults, she developed a map - a theory of evolving structures - which charted his journey from the chaos and confusion of his first moments, to a way he could think about, organize and relate to his world and the people in it.

She outlined a theory to describe developmental events which take place originally at a very early stage in human life - the first few months. This theoretical structure has proven highly effective in understanding the behaviour and disturbances of older children and adults. But because it concerns some very elusive concepts - particularly in relation to the very earliest experiences in the first couple of months in an infant's life - it is difficult to elucidate this structure in ordinary language, without falling back on the theory itself. We can't *know* what infants think or feel; but we have theories about it based on the analysis of adults and older children, direct infant observation studies, philosophical studies of theories of mind, and more empirical infant studies. When reading what follows it is important to remember that

the words 'in Kleinian theory' should be understood to precede any statement about what infants feel, or what they do in their minds.

Klein used the term 'position' to make an important point: she wanted the
concept of positions to be understood differently from the concept of
'stages', such as Freud's oral, anal, phallic and genital stages which follow one
another in a regular sequence and which the healthy individual, for the most
part, passes through in sequence. In Kleinian theory, the paranoid-schizoid
position and the depressive position are, *and remain throughout*, the two
elemental structures of emotional life. They have their origin in early childhood, indeed, in the first months of life. But the term 'position' applies not
only to particular stages of infant development, it applies also to modes of
psychic functioning which last all through life. Each of the two positions has
its own characteristic anxieties, its own defence mechanisms and its own
type of object relations. Each describes an attitude of mind.

Klein's delineation of these different constellations is perhaps her greatest
gift to psychoanalysis. The concept of positions is itself a structure which
enables us to understand two basically different configurations of object
relations, the anxieties that arise from them, and the mechanisms used to
protect against such anxieties; and the differences between the two positions
can in fact be defined in the same terms. To be over-simplistic, a person in the
depressive position feels concern for and worry about damage to his objects
– his loved ones – in external reality and in his mind ('I was nasty and really
unkind to my mother this morning'); while a person in the paranoid-schizoid
position feels anxiety for himself: for his own safety ('My mother always
phones me up at the wrong time'). Thus, anxiety in the depressive position is
linked to guilt ('I feel really bad about how unkind I was to her; I'm sure she
was hurt'); while anxiety in the paranoid schizoid position is persecutory
('I'm sure she hates me now and will probably tell my sister about it'). And
while someone whose state of mind is more characteristic of the depressive
position can view his loved ones as whole people, with their own real good
and bad qualities, it is characteristic of people in the paranoid schizoid
position that they see other people as being either perfect, and therefore
acceptable, or very persecuting, and therefore entirely unacceptable.

It is easy to understand, then, why the paranoid-schizoid position seems
to play the role of the ugly stepsister of the two positions. There is a powerful
tendency to see paranoid-schizoid phenomena as, at best, ill and, at worst,
immoral. The paranoid-schizoid position is where we feel we shouldn't be,
and a kind of morality can attach itself to the notion of paranoid-schizoid vs.
depressive phenomena, a morality which is misplaced and is based on a
misunderstanding. In fact, for all their differences, the two positions are also
on a continuum – a continuum of increasing integration, in which each
achievement is based on and dependent on the achievements that came

before. And in the development of the individual, the ability to fully establish the proper bi-partite paranoid-schizoid position is the first, and a fundamental, developmental achievement.

Three assumptions basic to Kleinian theory

The paranoid-schizoid position is the earliest, and for three or four months the only means by which the small infant can structure his experiences. In order to understand what this entails, it is necessary to take account of three assumptions basic to Kleinian theory. These are *the ubiquitousness of unconscious phantasy*, *the infant's inherent capacity to relate to objects*, and *the duality of the life and death instincts*.

Unconscious phantasies

Klein assumed that from the moment of our birth, all our experiences are accompanied by unconscious phantasies (see Chapter 2). These phantasies, specific to the individual, are ubiquitous, and are constantly active in everyone. They are nothing more or less than the life of the unconscious mind, and they are the representations of all an individual's experiences, internal, external, physical or mental. They are primitive and in some cases permanent phantasies which the ego has about itself and its relation to its internal objects, and they become the basis of the structure of the personality.

The relationship to objects

According to Kleinian theory, infants relate to objects in reality and in phantasy from birth onwards (see Chapter 8). Klein insisted that the smallest baby experiences both hatred and real love for its object, and furthermore that this love is directed not just at the feeding breast but very soon at the mother herself, however vaguely perceived and with whatever distortions. Her point is that the infant is innately constituted to turn towards his mother, in love and in hate. This leads us to consider what Kleinians mean by a 'good object'. It is not a mysterious term, nor a sentimental one, nor an idealizing one. A 'good object' simply means that person whom the infant begins to expect will satisfy it. Klein thought that the expectation of a 'good' object, a someone who will both satisfy the infant's hunger and be the recipient of his loving feelings, is constitutional: that infants are born expecting to find such a person. In fact, recent infant studies confirm such a hypothesis (Bower, 1977; Carpenter, 1975; Sander, 1969; all in Petot, 1991, pp. 248-51). It is important to understand that what is meant by a 'good' object is an object felt to be good by the life-loving aspects of the subject. It is not an objective statement about the goodness or otherwise of a mother, or father, or psychoanalyst.

The life and death instincts

Kleinian theory is a theory of instinctual dualism; it is about the contradictions in our nature. Following Freud, Klein maintained that from birth the infant is endowed with life instincts and death instincts; how these are bound, deployed, deflected, projected, re-introjected – how conflicts between life and death instincts, or love and hatred, are dealt with – may be said to be the determining characteristic of an individual's object relations and personality. The newborn infant, then, according to Klein, is beset from birth by powerful impulses in conflict with one another – impulses which, on the one hand, propel it towards life and the recognition of objects, the perception of reality, the organization of experience; and, on the other hand, invade it with threats of dissolution, of chaos, of disorder. This conflict, between his innate wish to live, to connect, to thrive, and his innate tendencies to dissolve, to disconnect, to not-be, create anxieties within the smallest infant. Anxiety, even at this earliest stage, is fear of the death instinct inside.

These three concepts relate to each other: the infant's impulses to love and to hate are always experienced in terms of his unconscious phantasies about his relationships with his objects.

The infant has an ego from the beginning. It is rudimentary at first, but it is present from birth. This ego has various abilities from birth, but they are uncoordinated and unintegrated. The integration of the ego, its cohesion and coordination, come about through experiences which enable it to incorporate and identify with a good object. Essentially what this means is that the small baby can achieve a representation of itself – a picture of itself – only by forming a picture of itself modelled on that of the person it loves.

In order for the infant to deal with, on the one hand, powerful internal conflicts (conflicts between life and death instincts which create often overwhelming anxieties), and, on the other hand, the frustrations and demands of external reality, its ego must gradually strengthen and develop. Random sensations, perceptions and impulses must begin to become structured and comprehensible – this requires an ego of some strength and cohesion. The first task for the infant, then, is the organization and structuring of its ego, and the organization of its experience, so that it can gradually begin more or less accurately to perceive and manage internal and external events (see Chapter 11). These two processes – the organization and structuring of its ego, and the organization of its experience – are mutually interdependent and dialectically related.

Capable, it will be remembered, of perceiving and responding to objects from the beginning of life, the infant is also capable from the beginning of experiencing events, and therefore objects felt to be attached to them, as good (e.g. a warm full tummy) or bad (hunger pains, colic). The infant begins internalizing, incorporating, identifying with good experiences from the first: he takes them into his ego. Gradually, his ego coheres around these repeatable, eventually expectable experiences of his good object. *In other words, the infant gradually begins to have an unconscious sense of himself, and his sense of himself is largely based on and dependent upon his sense of his good object in good experiences.*

The infant, then, must therefore protect his sense of his good object, on which his growing sense of himself is based, from his own feelings of hatred and rage – his innate hatred as well as the rage growing out of inevitable frustrations. He must also protect his developing ego from the dangers presented by his death instinct – the danger of fragmentation and dissolution. He must, in other words, safeguard his mind to allow it to develop and strengthen. The complex psychological structure which enables him to do this is called the paranoid-schizoid position.

In the paranoid-schizoid position, the infant divides his perception of his experiences into two categories, in such a way as to minimize his anxieties. He divides his world into 'good' which he attempts to possess and to be, and 'bad' which he tries to get rid of and locate outside himself, in his object. 'Good' for the infant thus equals 'Me', and it is made up of good object/good me. 'Bad' equals 'Not me', and it is made up of bad object/bad me. The mechanisms used by the infant to create this bi-polar world are *splitting* and *projection*. Splitting refers to the way the infant (and later in development the child and the adult) splits his picture of his object (one mother) into two felt-to-be-completely-different objects: a good one, and a bad one. The concept of splitting refers to an unconscious phantasy in the mind of the subject – unconsciously, in his mind, he splits the qualities of the single object and divides them between two or more objects.

An example of the use of the mechanism of splitting in an adult patient will help to illustrate what it means for someone to 'split his object':

A 35-year-old man had recently begun analysis. In the first few weeks of the analysis he referred several times to his analyst as an 'old woman' or a 'very old woman'; when, for instance, he spoke about the slippery path to the consulting room, he mentioned that the analyst, 'a very old woman', would need to be careful walking down the path. On an evening during the third weekend break of this new analysis, the analyst was in a large theatre when she realized that her patient was in the lobby of that same theatre. The analyst was talking with several friends; the patient walked past her, looked straight at her, stopped and looked more closely for ten or fifteen seconds, and then moved on, came back and looked closely again and then left. In the Monday session, the patient reported that on the weekend he had been in a theatre lobby and had seen a very attractive middle-aged woman, who looked a lot like his analyst, but much younger. It occurred to him that his analyst might have been a good-looking woman many years ago. From there the patient went on to talk about his sexual experiences when he was a young man, including some visits to a prostitute.

Obviously, the patient had *split* his perception of his analyst: his one analyst in his mind had become two people in his mind. There was his analyst, who is old and frail and certainly not at all a sexual object, and there was a middle-aged woman in the theatre who was attractive and gave rise to sexual fantasies. He had 'split his object', probably in order to keep his sexual feelings as far away as possible from his picture of his analyst as a maternal figure.

But he had done more than that. In order to split his object, the patient had also to split his own ego. That is, he had to disconnect two parts of his experience from each other. He couldn't put together the part of him that recognized his analyst in the theatre with the part of him that insisted that his analyst was a very old woman. To have brought these two perceptions together would have required that he bring together the two ideas 'analyst' and 'attractive woman', and for him these two ideas were not compatible. And so he created a split in his ego. This is an important point, because it emphasizes that one cannot, in fact, split one's objects without causing a split in one's ego. And a split in one's ego implies a reduction in ego capacities, a reduction in the capacity to think clearly.

The second of the two basic defence mechanisms in the paranoid-schizoid position is *projection*, and it goes along with and accompanies splitting. When the infant, and later the adult, splits off his own unwanted impulses, he projects them outside himself, into his object. Freud thought that the infant deals with his death instinct by 'deflecting' it, and Klein agreed with him. Deflecting his death instinct means that the infant *splits off* his death instinct and *projects it* outside himself – he experiences the danger as coming from outside him, and not inside him in his very self. He attributes aggression, danger, hatred to someone else. So splitting here refers to a split in the infant's perception of himself – he splits himself into a loving self and a hating self and gets rid of his perception of the hating self by attributing his own dangerous violent feelings to someone else – he *projects* them into his object and believes they are true of his object and not of himself. Thus the object is perceived as dangerously persecuting.

Another example, this time from the analysis of a woman adult patient, may illustrate the process of projection:

This patient was a 35-year-old writer who had come to analysis because she was worried about not being able to hold on to any confidence about her work or her relationships.

One day she came to her session and, after an initial reluctance, told me that an important literary critic had written to her, full of admiration for her work, and wanting to help her get published in what she referred to as 'a very well known' literary magazine. She reported that when she got the letter she was delighted, but she immediately began to feel worried: maybe he, the critic, didn't really like her work but had been pushed to write to her because he knows her boss; how unfair it is that her work gets a chance to be recognized when so many better writers go unnoticed because they don't have the connections she does, etc. etc. As she spoke, I noticed among other things that she was very deliberately not telling me either the name of the 'famous' critic, or the name of the 'famous' magazine. I carefully pointed this out to her, and said I didn't want her to tell me now, but I wanted to draw our attention to the fact that she didn't mention any names. After a moment she said that she was aware that she wasn't telling me the details, because as she'd begun to speak she'd had the thought that I would think she was boasting, that she had gotten too self-confident, and that I would want to bring her down.

We began to be able to see the degree to which she can split off her own self-destructive attacks on her achievement and attribute them to someone else, in this case her analyst. She projected her destructive feelings into me, and felt them to belong to me. (In fact of course this process was more complicated. This patient had an internal object which persecuted her and begrudged her any success; this internal object was linked with a picture of her mother altered by the patient's projections into the mother. It was this internal object, itself a result of perceptions, projections and introjections, that the patient had projected into me.)

Splitting, then, refers both to the splitting of the object into Good and Bad, and the splitting of the ego, also often into good and bad. *Projection* refers to the way certain qualities, characteristics or feelings which belong originally to the self, are disowned by the ego and attributed to someone else. [(This entire process, in which unbearable aspects of the self are split off and projected into another person who is then felt to be like (identified with) those split-off qualities, later became known as *projective identification*; see Chapter 9)]

Sometimes the aspects of the self which are projected are the felt-to-be-bad, felt-to-be-dangerous aspects – like in the clinical example above – where destructiveness is projected into an other because it is felt to be so dangerous and destructive inside the self. But often someone projects his or her good, valuable qualities into his or her object. This might seem more difficult to understand, but in fact it is a common event. If I have little confidence in my ability to stand up for something I believe in, say, because I know how subject I am to inner doubts and anxieties, I may project leadership, strength, fortitude, bravery into my teachers, or my seniors; I allow them to take over abilities which I feel I cannot take care of in myself. Or if I am unconsciously afraid to use my intelligence because I am (also unconsciously) aware of how triumphant and superior I might become, I may find that I become a little stupid, or awkward, and attribute great intelligence to someone else, a brother perhaps, whom I trust to take care of this quality.

Projecting good qualities can serve an important function: to project loving feelings into someone is to allow them to be seen to be loving. The positive effect this can have can be observed in a mother and her newborn –

the infant smiles at his mother, attributing to her his own loving feelings. Mother, delighted at being looked at lovingly, smiles back, with her own loving feelings. A benign circle is in process. But if projection of goodness is excessive, the infant, and later the adult, can feel depleted of anything good in himself, and becomes overly dependent on an idealized object.

> Mrs K, a married woman with two children, reported feeling desperately empty and lifeless every time her mother, who lived in a town some miles away, left after a visit. She could only comfort herself by thinking about past experiences with the mother: the mountains where they had been together when Mrs K was a child, what the mother had cooked for her, and so on. For some days after each visit Mrs K was without energy or enthusiasm; she felt, she said, as if all the life had left her.

In these early months, the infant's experiences are extreme, intense and absolute. Because he doesn't yet have the capacity of memory, events are timeless: Now is forever, there is no sense of time passing, no memory of yesterday or an hour ago, no expectation of later. Now is all there is. In these circumstances, Bad is perceived as unmitigated Bad – there is at first no useful memory of Good to modify it. The bad persecuting object has every bad experience projected into it, and it contains, in the infant's phantasies, everything which hurts him: everything that tears at him in hunger, or irritates his skin, or makes his tummy burn, or terrifies him. Against this persecuting object the infant employs all the forces he has available to him in phantasy: he imagines he tears at it, urinates on it, evacuates bad feelings into it, bites it to pieces. Once it is felt to contain everything bad in the world, no attack is too extreme for it. And, of course, it is then felt to attack back with re-doubled force in revenge. It is important to remember that these attacks all take place *in phantasy*; when, for example, the infant's skin is burning from nappy rash, and he imagines a bad mother is hurting him, he *phantasizes* that his angry screams and, coming at the same time, his urination, attack her and burn her. He unconsciously imagines this; it is part of his *unconscious phantasy* of what is happening.

However destructive these phantasized attacks are, in fact the most powerful weapon the infant has in his armament is a phantasy in the negative mode: a *negative hallucination*, a denial. In a negative hallucination, the object is annihilated from the infant's mind. It is not thought of. It has been made not to exist. The violence of this process is ferociously destructive; it wipes out the object from existence (Freud, 1901; Klein, 1946).

There is a passage in *Swann's Way* in which Proust describes Mlle Vinteuil deliberately and horribly attacking her recently dead father by licentiously performing all kinds of sexual acts with her lesbian lover directly in front of her father's photograph. Proust remarks that, of course, by doing so the daughter is only demonstrating her involvement with and attachment to her dead father, even if the involvement is an angry one. The ultimate attack, he points out, would have been to completely ignore the father, to have no thought of him, for him not to exist in her mind at all, 'that *indifference* ... which, whatever other names one gives it, is the most terrible and lasting form of cruelty' (Proust, 1981).

In order to understand that this concept of denial, or negative hallucination, is about violent destruction, it is necessary to have a picture of the mind in which unconscious phantasies always exist. One of the infant's earliest means of comforting himself in the face of frustration is the capacity to phantasize an endlessly good and gratifying object. This is an object that will always be there, will always be full of goodness, will always exist for and only for the infant. It thus creates no anxiety. This is a phantasy of hallucinatory gratification – gratification by a perfect object. But in order omnipotently to maintain such a phantasy, the infant must *deny* the existence of a bad and frustrating object. This can only be accomplished by means of some violent phantasy. And this denial of the existence of the bad object can only be accomplished by destroying, by splitting off from awareness, the part of the self that relates to the bad object, fearing it and hating it. And as with all such splits in the ego, this leads to impoverishment in the capacity to think and to feel.

And of course the bad, persecuting object, banished to some dark non-being, can suddenly and without warning emerge into being again. The persecutor could, it is felt, arrive unannounced and without warning at any time, and its attacks must therefore constantly be pre-empted.

> Ms L, a 23-year-old woman in analysis, who wants desperately to maintain a good relationship with me, constantly interrupts her speech to me with, 'I know you'll say I'm silly,' or 'I can just imagine what you think about that.' She is continually on the look-out for an unexpected persecution.

It is precisely because of the terrifying qualities of the bad object, which contains all of the infant's own sadism, that the good mother must be experienced as Ideal – as unmitigated Good. The two polarities must be maintained in their extreme form – the Good, to keep it far away from the feelings about the Bad, must be felt to be not just good, it must be perfect and unassailable, and therefore untouchable by anything bad. This is because the infant needs to keep his good objects and his good self, which is still fragile, from being attacked by his dangerous impulses. *Idealization*, then, is a normal and necessary stage in early infant development. It enables the good object to be taken in and identified with – installed in the infant's ego – and protected from his attacks. It is this identification with the good (ideal) object which gives strength to his early sense of himself, gives him a sense of coherence, and helps the infant hold on from one good experience to another. As cognitive functions – especially memory and perception – improve with normal maturation, this developing self, identified with its good (ideal) object, will eventually allow the splitting to come together. Eventually 'ideal' will not be necessary – good will be good enough. But under difficult conditions in later life, as a growing child and as an adult, when good feelings about himself are threatened, and when his sense of his good objects is threatened, the person may turn to idealization again, temporarily or for an extended period.

> Mr D describes how when he was sent to boarding school at 11 he was horribly homesick and lonely for the first weeks, feeling that he was falling into 'a pit of loneliness and despair'. One day he saw a young girl in the school and 'fell in love' with her. From that moment on he felt better; he was able to get down to his studies and to excel in all his classes, because, although (and, in fact, because) he never spoke more than a word or two to her over the next seven years, he told himself that he was studying and working 'for her'.
>
> He had established an ideal object in his mind, which he could keep completely separated from his anger with his parents and his jealousy of his younger brother who was at home.

It is important to recognize that it is, in fact, within the paranoid-schizoid position that the good object is first introjected as a complete and in some sense whole object (1946, p. 297). This first internal good (ideal) object isn't true to the full reality of the external object – Mr D, for instance, had hardly spoken to his young muse – but it is whole in the sense of having qualities beyond the purely functional – the good object in the paranoid-schizoid position is loved not just because it feeds but because it inspires and is felt to return the infant's love. It is a whole object, not just a part-object.

Splitting and projection are the infant's first ego defence mechanisms – this means that they defend his ego – his sense of his self – against overwhelming anxiety and confusion. For the infant, the purpose of separating Good (Ideal) and Bad is to protect the developing ego and the good objects from the death instinct. Splitting between Good and Bad is thus in the service of the life instincts. The goal of the paranoid-schizoid position, and the defence mechanisms available within it, is the first and most basic structuring of the personality: the earliest organization of experience. It is the first step, the beginning, of coherence. In so far as it organizes the infant's world into two discrete categories: Good, and Bad; and so long as these categories are not either too weak or too rigidly maintained, splitting – that is bi-polar splitting – is a psychological achievement.

Problems in the achievement of healthy paranoid-schizoid bi-polarity

The dangers in the paranoid-schizoid position are twofold, and can be described as (a) an inability to establish real bi-polarity, or (b) a too rigid and too extreme bi-polarity.

The first danger is that, for a number of reasons, binary or bi-polar splitting is never properly established. This is the most serious of the two dangers: if no real dichotomy can be established between what is good and what is bad, then what is good is constantly threatened, and the results can be catastrophic for the ego. Faced with constant threats to itself and its good objects, the ego splits in a harmful and sometimes catastrophic way – it fragments itself into many bits, and then the bits themselves are violently projected.

The following clinical material illustrates the different kinds of splitting (I have used this material in another context):

In a Monday session, Mrs T spoke about her busy weekend, describing it as marvellously successful; she described how she had invited some juniors from her workplace to her home, and how they had been filled with envy about everything she had. She commented how difficult it must have been for them all to see how much she and her family have. Based on a great deal of material, I interpreted to her that when she described all this to me she thought that I, too, was like the struggling 'juniors', enviously watching her. And that I thought this was designed to protect her from what she otherwise might feel about the weekend break: how determined she was that she be the enviable centre of everything.

I was thus interpreting that she had projected her envy of her analyst (standing in the transference for her primary object) into the juniors and, in the session, into me. That is, she imagined me as envious, and wasn't at all aware of any envious feelings in herself - she had split off the part of herself capable of feeling envy, and had located (projected) it into me.

This interpretation seemed to allow her to take back the part of her which she had projected. Following this interpretation she was able to tell me more about the weekend. She told me that in fact she and her husband had had a terrible row about his not being more available to her, and she had shouted and screamed at him and hit him several times in front of the children. She was so angry that she had screamed at the children about how horrible their father was. The children were terribly upset. She commented sadly that these fights with her husband always seemed to happen in front of the children. (She was now no longer feeling like the enviable one, she was able to be aware of some very painful feelings.)

I interpreted to her that she was now more in touch with her rage with me on the weekend, for not being available to her, and I linked her attacks on her husband with this rage with me. She was listening to me, so I went on. I said I thought her furious fights had to be observed by her children because they, the children, had to be the observers of the violence of the sexual parents - a view of the parents originating in her own violent attacks on them. I said that while she insists that she feels nothing at all about my weekends, she was showing us that there is a child who is horrified and appalled and furious and disturbed at what parents are doing - but that it was not going to be experienced by her, it would have to be experienced by her children. I said she makes her children have this experience which she feels is unbearable for her.

I was thus interpreting a complex sequence of splits and projections. She split her objects: I was allowed to remain good in her mind, while her husband became intolerably bad. All the rage she felt for me was then directed at him. But she also used her children to carry projections of parts of herself - they had to be horribly, painfully aware of parents together in a terrible, violent way. (I thought that when, unconsciously, she imagined my weekend, and my being together with my husband, it was with such jealousy and violence that in her mind the couple could only come together in violence. The observation of all this had to be projected into her children, who were horrified and lonely.)

This interpretation came at the end of the session and I think confronted her with what she was doing to her children, and therefore with guilt. Her response was dramatic. On the following day the patient reported in her session that she had been in a terrible panic all night. She had suddenly become terrified of pollution: she thought there were particles of it in the air all around her; she was sure the pollution had got into the house and that there was poison everywhere. She was terrified about its effect on everyone.

I thought that she was telling me what she had done with the interpretation of the previous day. That session had centred on a report about her putting very painful, horrible feelings into her children, and today's session was about millions and millions of infinitesimal small particles which were poisoning her children and her husband and herself. I thought this was her way of dealing with the guilt she had been threatened with experiencing when she began to see what she was doing to her children, and behind that, to me in her mind. She had projected the poison into the atmosphere - but in millions of tiny fragments so that it was then felt to be coming at her from all directions. It was not experienced as coming from inside her but as coming from outside.

She had fragmented the dangerous guilty feelings into many bits and projected them outside.

This left her in a state of agitated panic; she was left temporarily unable to think about herself or her children or the situation. When I could show her how her mind had become split in many little pieces and projected into the atmosphere outside, she began to be able to think again.

This excessive splitting, often resulting from overwhelming persecutory anxiety, is very different from the binary differentiation we have been discussing. This kind of splitting into many bits is often referred to as fragmentation. It can lead to a terrifying sense of confusion and disintegration, a feeling of chaos and depersonalization. In its most extreme form it is linked with schizophrenic processes.

Splitting into many bits - fragmentation - occurs for a number of reasons, but *envy* is very often a powerful factor. The reason is this: in order to make the differentiation between good and bad which is necessary for proper binary splitting to take place, Good (or ideal) must be allowed to exist. If the infant's envious feelings are too powerful, he cannot permit the existence of goodness in his loved one; his awareness of having experienced its goodness provokes his envy of it, and makes him attack and try to destroy it. In this sense, envy is much more dangerous for the health of the individual than is sadism. One's loved one can recover from a sadistic attack; afterwards, powerful loving feelings towards her mean that confidence in the goodness of the loved object can be restored. But it is exactly the felt-to-be-goodness of the object which is under attack when the attacks are motivated by envy.

In the analysis of children and of adults it is terribly important to differentiate attacks on the analyst when she is felt to be bad (attacking, frustrating, depriving, misunderstanding) from attacks on the analyst precisely when she is felt to be good.

Binary splitting – splitting the object and the self into two distinct categories Good and Bad – organizes and structures what was previously chaotic experiencing; when it fails as a mechanism, chaos and confusion result. Confusion is, for Klein, the worst, most painful state of mind. It is the mind falling apart and falling into bits. It is also, paradoxically, the ultimate refuge when persecutory anxiety becomes too overwhelming to bear: the mind that could know the persecution dissolves itself.

Rigid and extreme bi-polarity

The other potential danger in the paranoid-schizoid position is that the two extremes become rigidly and impermeably separated. This is less dangerous than the catastrophe of confusional states, but it severely limits development, and prevents the person from moving into the depressive position.

When splits are rigidly maintained, objects can never grow in resilience, and the personality remains brittle and inflexible. In the paranoid-schizoid position, as we have seen, the good object never has to be recognized as separate from the self; the good object *is* the good self, from whom all good experiences come. It is not the same object as the bad object, from whom all bad experiences come, and who appears the moment the good object disappears. These are two distinct objects. In the paranoid-schizoid position there is good mother, who belongs entirely to me and who brings me endless pleasure. But the moment I feel distress, there is no good mother, I am completely in the presence of the bad mother who is persecuting me. These are states of mind which fluctuate rapidly.

To perceive the object more realistically I must recognize that the mother who isn't there when I need her is the same mother who comes and brings me comfort: the mother I hate is the same mother as the mother I love. And I have to recognize that she is not Me, she does not always belong to me. This requires an acceptance of a painful, sometimes too painful, reality: that I am dependent on an object which is not Me, and which is independent of me. And that I have attacked and damaged, and continue to attack and damage, the very person I love and need.

These realizations are the beginning of ambivalence (having mixed feelings about someone) and of guilt. And they already exist, though fleetingly, and powerfully defended against, in the paranoid-schizoid position.

I said at the beginning of this chapter that the paranoid-schizoid position can be differentiated from the depressive position on the basis of the anxieties characteristic of each; and that while persecution is characteristic of the paranoid-schizoid position, guilt is more characteristic of the depressive position (see Chapter 3). Of course, by and large this is true; and in fact the depressive position is defined by the capacity to bear painful guilt about one's attitude towards and treatment of one's loved ones. But guilt exists in rudimentary and either fragmentary or projected forms in the paranoid-schizoid position; Klein is clear about this (1957), and it is evident from the work of her followers. For example, Rosenfeld described a schizophrenic patient who attacked a nurse in the hospital where he was being treated:

> He attacked Sister X suddenly, while he was having tea with her and his father, hitting her hard on the temple. She was affectionately putting her arms round his shoulders at the time. The attack occurred on a Saturday, and I found him silent and defensive on Monday and Tuesday. On Wednesday he talked a little more. He said that he had destroyed the whole world and later on he said 'Afraid.' He added, 'Eli' (God) several times. When he spoke he looked very dejected and his head drooped on his chest. I interpreted that when he attacked Sister X he felt he had destroyed the whole world and he felt only Eli could put right what he had done. He remained silent. After continuing my interpretations by saying that he felt not only guilty but afraid of being attacked inside and outside, he became a little more communicative. He said 'I can't stand it any more.' Then he stared at the table and said, 'It is all broadened out, what are all the men going to feel?' I said that he could no longer stand the guilt and anxiety inside himself and had put his depression, anxiety and feelings, and also himself into the outer world. As a result of this he felt broadened out, split up into many men, and he wondered what all the different parts of himself were going to feel. (Rosenfeld, 1952, p. 79)

Rosenfeld's material demonstrates several aspects of paranoid-schizoid phenomena: the patient attacks the nurse and then feels not only persecution but also guilt, and depression. But the material makes it clear that he cannot bear the feelings of guilt and depression, and that he very quickly fragments his awareness of them, projecting into the resulting 'many men' his own capacities to think and to feel. As a result he is left not knowing what he feels – depersonalized and confused.

It is clear, then, that fleeting perceptions of reality, and fleeting intim-
ations of guilt cannot be long tolerated in the paranoid-schizoid position;
they are annihilated or fragmented or projected. But it is important to understand that they exist as fugitive perceptions and that their denial or projection brings consequent persecutory anxiety. In normal development, as the
ego strengthens, the reality of ambivalence, the pain of guilt, and the loss of
narcissistic omnipotence will be gradually more tolerable. When such reality
cannot be faced then the gradual integration of good and bad, inner and
outer, me and not-me cannot take place. In these circumstances, the splits are
widened, the dichotomies strengthened and made more rigid. In fact,
throughout life, when guilt feels too intense to bear, an individual will return
to the rigidity and safety of the paranoid-schizoid position, where he can tell
the Good Guys from the Bad Guys and maintain with absolute certainty that
he is on the side of the Good.

CHAPTER 4

The depressive position

JANE TEMPERLEY

In 1935, with her paper 'A contribution to the psychogenesis of manic-depressive states', Klein began a theoretical reorganization of her insights in terms of 'positions'. A position refers to 'a state of organization of the ego – the nature of the internal object relations and the nature of the anxiety and the characteristic defences'. In the 1935 paper she refers to manic and paranoid positions as well as to the depressive position, but in her eventual formulation there are two positions, the paranoid-schizoid and the depressive.

The paranoid-schizoid position precedes the depressive position developmentally and although Klein describes the six-month baby as struggling with the depressive position, the oscillation between these positions continues throughout life.

Klein is an instinct theorist in that she held that from the beginning of life the infant has to contend with strong instinctual impulses towards life and towards death. In this she continued Freud's last and contentious restatement – in *Beyond the Pleasure Principle* (1920a) – of the instinctual conflicts governing human subjectivity. These drives are experienced in terms of unconscious phantasies involving the subject (his ego) in relation with an object, towards whom the drive is expressed. The hungry baby searches for a satisfying breast or rages at one that frustrates him.

For fear of the death instinct which threatens it from within and because of its own initial frailty, the early ego protects itself with the mechanisms of splitting and projection. As described in the previous chapter, it splits off what feels disturbing and dangerous in itself and projects these aspects of itself into the object. It also splits the object, seeing its gratifying aspects as ideal and its frustrating aspects as hostile. At this stage the object is in any case apprehended only in part, as a satisfying or frustrating breast, for instance, rather than as a whole person. The infant seeks to strengthen its inner world both by splitting off and projecting its disturbing aspects into external objects and by introjecting into itself the part objects it has idealized. In this way it seeks to protect itself against its primary anxiety which is for its own survival in the face of internal and external persecutors (see Chapter 3).

The transition to the depressive position involves a gradual integration both of the ego and of the object. With the maturation of the perceptual apparatus the child's capacity to modify his phantasies by comparing them with reality usually reduces anxiety. The internalization of good experiences and good objects reassures him about his inner state and he has less need to project. Because he feels less threatened by objects made bad by his projections, he feels less aggressive towards them and in turn he feels stronger and more whole because less impoverished by what in himself he had split off and lodged in those around him. He has less need to keep either himself or his object split. He is more able to recognize that the mother who was the idealized source of all life and goodness is also the mother who was previously experienced as the attacked and attacking frustrator from whom it was not safe to receive succour. She becomes an integrated figure with positive and negative features, towards whom the child feels ambivalence, both love and hatred.

As the child withdraws his projections, he becomes increasingly aware of his own mixed nature and of the tension that exists within him between his loving and destructive impulses. Since it is no longer a bad 'other' who is felt to be responsible for the aggression he has projected into the world around, the child begins to recognize his own responsibility and to experience guilt. This capacity to recognize and bear guilt is one of the reasons for Klein's choosing the term 'depressive' for this position.

The reduced use of projection and the greater integration of both the ego and the object leads to a more pronounced sense of separateness and of the infant's dependence on a separate other person. In the paranoid-schizoid position, Bion has remarked that there is no sense of an absent good object – the infant is either in the presence of a good object or, if the mother is unavailable, it is in the presence of a bad object. With the depressive position the child becomes aware that it does not control or possess the good object but needs it and can miss and pine for it in its absence. The child feels loss and mourning for a good object, rather than denial or betrayal by what is felt to be a bad object. Because of this new sense of its dependence on the object and of the dangers to the object from the child's own destructiveness, this stage is characterized by concern for the object. It is also marked by the development of the desire to repair and restore the object which the child fears it has damaged by its attacks. The capacity for reparation is one of the most powerful manifestations of the life instinct.

One of the earliest and most celebrated pieces of infant observation was Freud's account (1920a) of his little grandson's game with the cotton reel, throwing it into his crib and then retrieving it. Freud recognized that the child was trying to come to terms with his feelings of losing his mother (when she went out), missing her and then joyfully recovering her.

Freud had earlier, in *Mourning and Melancholia* (1915b), described how this process of negotiating loss can miscarry with dire consequences for the subject's inner life. Where the feelings towards the disappointing figure are predominantly hateful she is not missed and pined for but unconsciously attacked and then set up within the internal world as a bad object. The self-torment so characteristic of melancholia is in a Kleinian perspective the continuing relationship within the self of the subject's failure to negotiate the depressive position, to do what Freud's little grandson was doing, to find a way to recover loving feelings towards someone who had hurt or left him. What Abraham and Klein added to Freud's momentous understanding of melancholia was that in mourning too there is an internalization of a relationship. The mourner, originally the child who is capable of sustaining or recovering his sense of loving and therefore missing his absent mother, installs within himself a valued and sustaining figure who gives him inner strength. In Klein's words the child who was originally inside the mother now feels he has the mother within him.

The recognition of separateness and dependence and of vulnerability to loss involves negotiating the object's relationship with others, with siblings and especially the parents' relationship to each other. Klein maintained that the working through of the depressive position and of the Oedipus Complex were facets of the same process.

A similar relinquishment of control and recognition of separateness and difference is needed in the creative use of symbols. Segal (1957) has elucidated how the symbol, the symbolizer and the symbolized need their autonomous qualities freed from the projective identification which causes psychotics to confuse the symbol with what is symbolized. The ability to use symbols is an achievement of the depressive position and liberates the user from the concreteness of psychotic thinking (see Chapter 10).

These processes in relation to the external object are accompanied by and in constant interaction with the state of the subject's internal objects. Positive experiences with the external objects are introjected and modify bad internal objects and these more benign internal objects are in turn projected on to the external world which is perceived in a more positive light. This in turn may elicit a warmer response, resulting in a benign self-reinforcing cycle. A malignant self-reinforcing cycle may also develop.

The primary anxiety of the depressive position is for the state of the good internal object on which the subject's well-being is felt to depend in the same way as in the external world the child depends on the parents. A particular instance of this dependence on, and concern with, the state of an internal object is the relationship to the superego (see Chapter 8). Where the object that has been introjected is felt to be severe or injured and reproachful the subject's mental state is dominated by guilt and a sense of inadequacy. He seeks to satisfy or repair the internal object and if he is not successful his state is that of melancholia.

For Klein, the working through of the depressive position and the establishment of a good internal object were crucial for mental health. The frustrations and losses of life and the constant threat from destructive sources within the personality make the depressive position an achievement that is repeatedly lost and in need of re-establishing. She described the work of mourning which is required with every major loss and disappointment as 'rebuilding with anguish the inner world'. This is particularly difficult where the depressive position has been precariously established in the first place and leaves the personality in danger of regression to the defences of the paranoid-schizoid position or to undue mobilization of a defence more specific to the depressive position, mania.

Klein described how the process of mourning, whether for an actual death or for other losses and disappointments, involves a loss of the sense of having an internal good object. The mourner may for a time feel triumphantly oblivious towards an internal object whose importance is denied (as in mania) or at the mercy of vengeful, or dead and dying objects within him. Gradually he may recover his good objects and this process of repeatedly re-negotiating the depressive position can lead to a strengthening and deepening of it that is recognizable in the emotional maturity and depth achieved by some older people. Elliot Jacques (1965) traced this re-working of the depressive position in the lives and work of great creative artists. In 'Death and the mid-life crisis' he suggests that in mid-life illusions of immortality need to be relinquished and a painful journey of self-exploration undertaken which can produce a more profound creativity.

The need to have a good object within one, to introject and indeed to incorporate it, as the baby originally incorporated what it received from the mother's breast, can be followed in the beliefs underlying the Christian service of Holy Communion. The Christian believes that in this ceremony he installs in his inner being a loved and loving protector (indeed an omnipotent one) who will sustain him in his struggles with the Devil, the representative of his own destructiveness and of the evil he may encounter in others. Loss of this divine object's good will is attributed to the believer's neglect of, and attacks upon, it and this loss results in guilt and intense fears of retaliation and Hell – an equivalent to the persecutory states suffered by severe melancholics. Though the ideal and omnipotent nature of the internal object that the Christian seeks to introject corresponds to the ideal and omnipotent figures of the paranoid-schizoid position, the yearning for a good internal object and the sense of responsibility, guilt and concern towards it belong to the depressive position. The central anxiety of the depressive position is about sustaining or recovering a good internal object.

A major defence against this anxiety is mania, a condition that often alternates with melancholia in a manner that has always interested clinicians. Klein, building upon Freud's and Abrahams' observations, saw that implicit in the excited omnipotence of manic states is a disparagement of the object. In the manic state the patient is no longer, as in the melancholic state, subject to the reproaches of a severe internal object. In phantasy he reduces his good internal objects to replaceable trivia that he can omnipotently control and simultaneously he rids himself of the more tormenting figures of the paranoid-schizoid phase. He is excitedly superior and condescending towards his object, triumphing over him and controlling him. In his racy grandeur he feels he has an abundance of everything and values nothing. There is a tremendous attack upon the psychic reality of his actual dependence on his internal and external objects. Their goodwill is wasted and destroyed with the result that once the mania has abated the internal objects are felt to be empty and damaged and melancholia reasserts itself. There is no real sense of guilt or recognition of the value of the object. Reparation where it is attempted has a magical, condescending quality that does not acknowledge what has been damaged and shows no real concern for the object.

Movement between the paranoid-schizoid and the depressive positions is illustrated in the behaviour of an adolescent girl at war with her parents and her teachers. Although intellectually able, she could not concentrate; she attacked and repulsed her parents when they attempted to help her and she insisted that the only solution was for her to change schools. Although the rows with her parents and the under-achievement continued at the new school she did get an A in one of her exams. The following scene occurred some weeks later. She and her mother were returning home by car. Her mother remarked that there was to be a meeting at the school for the girl and her parents to discuss her work. The girl reacted angrily, abused her mother and walked away from her as they left the car. She shouted at her mother that all her parents wanted was a model pupil. The mother noticed, when she entered the house, that the girl was sitting on the floor attempting to glue back on to her shoe the sole which had come apart. (Previously when this shoe needed repair she had tossed it to her father to get it mended.) The mother sat down beside her and said that she didn't want a model pupil but that they both knew her schooling was important and that she could do justice to her ability. The daughter then told her mother how bad she felt about herself, especially in relation to other pupils who had worked hard and well. The mother felt relieved, less injured and angry herself, and more aware of her love and concern to help. After they had sat together talking while the girl continued to repair her shoe, the mother, so used to being repulsed, enquired if the girl now wanted to be on her own. 'No,' was the reply, 'you can stay.'

Like her shoe, this girl is at first unable to function because of the splitting that she has used – partly in order to cope with the new challenges accompanying her adolescence. Troubled by her own sense of badness she had split this bad self off and projected it into her parents and the school. They were then experienced as tormentors and she felt that she must fight them off and protect herself. She also attributed to her parents the idealized expectations characteristic of a flight from extremely bad objects to the supposed protection of ideal objects – who then in their turn demand an ideal response – a model pupil. Along with these tormenting aspects of herself the girl also projected on to the parents more positive aspects of herself – her capacity to recognize the reality of her situation at school and to work on this. In throwing her broken shoe at her father she gave concrete expression to how she was violently projecting on to him her own capacity to work at her problems.

The transition came when she sat down and attempted to repair the shoe herself, indicating that she was beginning to repair the split within herself and with it the rift between herself and her parents. She was able to withdraw the 'badness' from her picture of her mother and to acknowledge it in herself. The mother, freed from the projection of her daughter's 'badness', was then experienced by both of them as a helpful figure, a good object, to whom the daughter could turn for strength in facing her difficulties. The girl no longer felt so extremely 'bad' that she could not face her regret and guilt at what she had done to her chances at school. She could, with her parents' help, begin to mend what she had damaged in her school work and in her relation to them. She became capable of reparation. Like her shoe she felt more whole and better able to cope with reality. Somewhat grudgingly, in this new state, she could acknowledge her dependence on her mother as a separate person – 'No, you can stay.'

Having established this more depressive position, this more integrated sense of herself and her object, she would doubtless lose it again, become once again split and paranoid, but she would be strengthened to recover herself and her access to good aspects of herself and of her objects (see Chapter 5).

In this vignette an important part was played by the girl's unconscious use of symbols. She worked upon her need to heal the split within her, via the medium of her broken shoe. It is a mark of the depressive position that the subject has sufficiently withdrawn projections of himself from his objects, human and material, to be able to make use of their actual characteristics for creative and communicative purposes. Someone more deeply in the paranoid-schizoid position might have felt his soul (his psyche) was so projectively identified with the sole of the shoe that he could not use it symbolically to communicate within himself and to the mother his wish to put things right.

The incident also illustrates the constant interaction between internal and external objects. In her split, paranoid state of mind the girl's projection of her bad self on to the school and her parents did at times engender in them the anger and retaliation she feared. Their angry state was then introjected, confirming and augmenting her inner sense of persecution. A self-reinforcing malignant cycle between figures in the inner world and those in external reality then occurred. Through the shoe mending exchange, however, the girl was able to restore a more integrated sense of herself and her objects. She then found confirmation of this inner change in her actual mother's reaction, thereby installing within herself a renewed sense of a good helpful internal object capable of seeing both her strengths and weaknesses.

This girl was intensely dependent on her parents but, until the shoe incident, unable to acknowledge this and so to use their help. Prior to that exchange she controlled her parents and the school, keeping them as bad and useless. Interaction between her parents and the school she found threat-ening and she wanted to prohibit and attack it. Her dependence on her parents, though fiercely repudiated at a conscious level, was expressed through her ferocious watchful control of them as bad figures, carrying feared aspects of herself. This dependence differs from that which she begins to show when she turns to her mother and shares with her her distress about her self-destructiveness. The mother feels herself released from her daughter's hostility and freed as a separate person to be helpful. The girl's depressive dependence is consciously acknowledged and acts as a spur to reconciliation and repair.

In the shoe conversation she relinquished her attacking control of her parents and could let them have an intercourse with the school which she could allow to be benign. Movement from the paranoid-schizoid position to the depressive position is simultaneously a relinquishment of control of the parental couple (here the parents and the school), a recognition of their separateness and intercourse and a realization that in this shift a new freedom may be gained. Negotiation of the depressive position is intimately related to the working through of the Oedipus Complex (see Chapter 6). They are as parts of the same process.

I will now illustrate from two works of literature the effects upon the mental state of the relationship to internal objects. The books considered are William Styron's *Darkness Visible* and Jiri Weil's *Life with a Star*. Styron's book is an account of his own depressive breakdown, written in the hope of helping others struggling with suicidal melancholia. Weil's book is not overtly autobiographical but he shares with his hero the experience of being a Jew in Nazi Prague and finding a way to survive. Both books are accounts by men who survived sustained torment and a threat of annihilation and were helped to escape and recover. For Styron the torment and the threat of death were within himself. For Weil's narrator the threat and the persecution come from the external world, from the Nazi occupation. Both narrators have lost parents in childhood, Styron his mother, Weil's narrator both his parents.

Both narrators experience states of mind, in Weil's case hope, in Styron's case despair, which are intensely at variance with their external circumstances and with the attitudes of those around them. The manner in which Weil's narrator retains his sanity and his capacity to love indicates a securely established good internal object. Styron's narrative is of how failure to mourn his mother's death when he was a child left him prey, as he approached old age, to a melancholia which threatened him with suicide. In the course of his book he describes recovering his awareness of what his mother and her loss meant to him and how in that realization he began to recover some peace of mind. He regains her as a loved and missed internal object and in doing so rediscovers his wish to live. The determining factor in both narratives is the subjects' engagement with figures in their internal world that undermine or sustain them; whom they ignore or whom they acknowledge and miss. The crucial issue is the degree to which they have been able to establish and work through the depressive position.

Weil's narrator Roubicek is alone, afraid, hungry and cold, awaiting daily his summons to join a transportation to 'the East', to a death camp. He hates and fears the Nazis but sustains himself by imaginary dialogues with his absent lover Ruzena and by recalling happiness with her. Ruzena had urged him to flee Prague with her and he now regrets he did not heed her advice. At times he withdraws from the horrors of his actual experience into something akin to hallucinating her presence. This is not, however, just a withdrawal from reality to an idealized memory – insofar as she is a good internal object he remains capable of re-finding good objects where they exist in the world around him. He develops a friendship with a stray cat whom he calls Tomas. He sees in him a fellow sufferer, hungry, fearful, hunted, lonely. He feeds the cat what little he can spare – Jews are not allowed to keep pets – and eventually the animal comes to trust him, to greet him when he returns home and to share his sleeping bag. Tomas recovers his strength and his sleek healthy fur. Roubicek sees himself in Tomas and in his care of Tomas draws unconsciously on his own introjection of Ruzena (based on earlier introjections of good figures in his childhood) and identification with her. Addressing Tomas in the beginning of their friendship he says,

> 'You see, Tomas, I mean you no harm. You are beginning to believe me a little. But
> only a little. Wait, how can I explain what happiness is? Large bowls of milk for
> you, Tomas, with lots of cream floating on top and a roll spread with butter, raw
> liver and then to lie down in the sun and be warm and safe. All that exists. You
> must believe me.'

The imagery is evocative of the experience of being in the presence of a
good feeding mother. Roubicek tells Tomas, and himself, that though such a
good feeding mother is spectacularly absent in the world they share, she does
exist as a reality in his mind. The good internal mother is refound in his love
for his cat. Roubicek identifies Tomas with his doubting infantile self whom
he comforts as his own mother or Ruzena (his internal mother) are felt to
comfort him. As the soprano in Brahms' German Requiem sings, 'I who have
known a mother's love will comfort you.' In the experience of parenting or
offering care to someone else the carer often finds himself strengthened and
more secure in an internal recovery of closeness with what was best in his
own parents. He recovers and strengthens his sense of having helpful figures
within him and of being capable himself of goodness.

Roubicek, in his concern for Tomas, is also seeking to put right what he has
come to regret in relation to Ruzena. He did not heed her warnings about the
Nazis – he underestimated their destructiveness and this reflected an underesti-
mation of his own passive tendency to surrender to destructiveness in others.
The damage he did to Ruzena and to himself was in failing to take active steps to
counter both the deathliness of the Nazis and of his own near-fatal passivity
toward them. The book is an account of how he did eventually counter this
passive surrender in himself. He was able belatedly to make that much amends to
her even though his passive resignation to the forces of evil had lost him the life
he and Ruzena might have had together. In this particular sense Roubicek is not
merely the victim of a persecuting environment but of a passivity within himself
which has severely damaged his relationship with the person he loves most.

Roubicek has every reason to be paranoid – he is actively persecuted,
thrown off buses, debarred from most public places, made to wear a yellow
star. His sense of being persecuted is based on reality. His aunt and uncle by
contrast have reacted to the loss of their material possessions and the threat of
transportation and death by desperate projective mechanisms which lead
them to distort the reality around them. When Roubicek visits them they see
him as the greedy agent of their misfortunes. They accuse him of endangering
their lives by having a cat. When they are summoned for transportation they
refuse Roubicek's advice that they take warm clothes and food and choose
instead to leave them in the supposed safe keeping of predatory neighbours.
They reproach and accuse Roubicek. Because of their frightened and

desperate resort to splitting and projection they are unable to recognize the reality of Roubicek's helpfulness or of their neighbours' greed. Roubicek has become a bad figure for them and the neighbours good ones. Splitting and projection have radically and tragically distorted their perceptions of reality.

Roubicek survives because he can sustain a good internal object and strengthen it by what he introjects of his loving relation to Tomas. He does not distort reality by massive projection and this enables him to recognize a quality in a chance encounter that leads him to get to know and trust Joseph Materna. Materna, whose name has obvious associations with motherliness, belongs to a working-class resistance movement. Roubicek becomes an occasional visitor to Materna's house where Materna's mother feeds him and where Materna and his friends hold discussions. Materna suggests that Roubicek choose not to accept his transportation summons but go into hiding, which his group will arrange. Weil describes how difficult it is for Roubicek to accept the struggle and the danger that Materna's offer will involve. His cat has been shot and he has news that Ruzena too has been shot. To resist the Nazis – the death instinct – seems too difficult. His fellow Jews deplore those among them who complicate their relations with the Nazis by attempting escape, even by suicide. He is troubled by guilt. Some other Jew would have to take his place on the transport and he feels himself responsible. He is also afraid for his rescuers – realistically because of the reprisals they would risk. Some of this guilt has the hallmark of melancholia – he doubts his worthiness to be saved. He has to some extent introjected the Nazi view of his worthlessness and badness. Some of his fellow Jews have done this to such an extent that they accuse Jews who thwart the Nazis of giving Jews a bad name. This attitude now introjected has become a deadly superego with which he has to struggle. His reservations on behalf of his would-be rescuers do have in addition an appropriate concern for them that is characteristic of the depressive position.

Roubicek's misgivings about availing himself of Materna's offer indicate that he had to struggle with the omnipotence characteristic of severe depressive states. In these states the superego attributes blame and guilt of an omnipotent kind to the sufferer. Roubicek was not completely at the mercy of such an internal object. He was evidently able to appreciate that guilt and responsibility for what his rescuers might suffer lay primarily with the Nazis and that his rescuers were free agents. Where there is concern for the object but it still has some of the uncompromising qualities of ideal or persecuting objects of the paranoid-schizoid position, guilt too has omnipotent qualities. Children of divorcing parents, for instance, may hold themselves, consciously or unconsciously, responsible and only later and with help modify their guilt so that they can recognize that, though they regret their own part in what happened, they can realistically apportion responsibility to their parents. The severe internal objects to which the ego is subject in the early stages of the depressive position become modified, gentler and more realistic.

This book is an account of a terrible experience in the real world, of the persecution and horrors associated with wearing a stigmatizing badge, of life with a star. At another level it is an account of how Roubicek drew on an extraordinary capacity within him to sustain a star, the light of a good object he had known and knew how to recover and which enabled him to choose life.

One night he is on duty at the Jewish community headquarters and looks down from a balcony on the Jewish quarters of the city:

> Below me I saw the district as if it were in a deep black chasm and called in vain to the Lord. Now it seemed even smaller and more huddled in the dark poverty of its junkyard. It no longer belonged to the world. It was simply suffered to exist ... I looked at the rooftops so as not to look into an even deeper chasm but they too seemed to writhe with pain. I turned away from the black chasm and looked at the stars. They were shining brightly in the summer night. They were cold, indifferent but they shone over the whole city including this district, crouched under blows. 'I must look only at them,' I told myself. 'It's a pity I didn't see them earlier. I won't be alone any more when I think of them. They belong to me and have always belonged to me. Nobody can take them away from me.'

Here he contemplates despair, equating the district that no longer belongs to the world and is simply suffered to exist with his own tormented, rubbished state. He is close to the chasm of melancholia where no Lord, not even an idealized internal object, will hear him. He turns away and recovers his lasting good objects, felt to be cold and indifferent at this moment, but a presence that protects him from loneliness and inner persecution. When he recovers his awareness of the stars he regains a relationship within himself that strengthens him to cope with the external 'blows' under which perhaps he doesn't have to 'crouch'.

Styron's book is an account of a severe melancholia where his mental state was such a 'district as if it were in a deep black chasm and called in vain on the Lord'. 'Darkness visible' is Milton's description of Hell.

Styron, when he became ill, was a very successful writer with a staunch wife and no external cause for depression. He suspects, however, that the alcohol to which he had recently become allergic may have been protecting him for years from knowledge of his true state. The melancholia struck when he had just turned 60, a late mid-life crisis that marks the passage from the prime of life towards old age and the inevitability of death.

He begins the book with an extended account of an event that occurred as the melancholia was establishing its hold on him. He had been awarded a prestigious and lucrative French literary prize and, despite his depressed state, was in Paris to receive it. The widow of the distinguished man who established the award had arranged a luncheon in his honour to follow the prize-giving. Styron with difficulty coped with receiving the award but then greatly offended his hostess by announcing that he had made another lunch appointment. He then did accept her invitation but later in the day managed to drop the cheque on the floor and barely retrieve it.

This incident, given in much more detail than any other social exchange in the book, has evidently a significance for his account. Indeed, in an Author's Note, he regrets its omission from the text originally published by *Vanity Fair*. It was 'a trip which had special significance for me in terms of the depressive illness from which I had suffered'. He is in a mental state where he finds himself aggressively rejecting what a feeding and appreciative older woman is offering him. His behaviour transforms her from a benign figure into one who is injured and reproachful. The incident deserves its place in his account because it describes how Styron's inner world has become so bankrupt and tormented by reproach.

At this stage he makes no reference at all to the fact that his mother died when he was still a child. Indeed his researches into the meaning of melancholia, though far-reaching, make minimal reference to the extensive literature linking it to loss and especially to maternal loss in childhood. Freud famously remarked that the melancholic, unlike the mourner, does not know what it is that he has lost. Styron for much of his account seems to have overlooked his childhood bereavement as he overlooked his French hostess's lunch invitation and cheque. He also overlooks Freud's *Mourning and Melancholia*, while eagerly re-instating the term melancholia as more apt than 'depression'. This capacity to dismiss what is highly relevant in his life and reading may also have operated at the time of his mother's death. Did he, like many a bereft child, feel that his mother had dropped and lost interest in him and then, in his pain, identify with her, dropping her and withdrawing interest and meaning from her and her loss? His near rejection of his patroness's meal and his dropping of her cheque would then be an enactment of his identification with the dead mother who, he felt, discarded and dropped him. Symbolically he reverses his childhood experience. It is now he who punishes and dismisses the woman who fed and appreciated him.

What he has introjected is a mother of no significance, offering nothing of value, fit only to die. He has then unconsciously identified with this internal mother, fit only for suicide. There is no sense, as with Roubicek, of an internal dialogue with someone missed and valued. Instead the dialogue seems to be one of reproach, the deserted child robbing the feeding mother of significance and she in turn reproaching him.

Styron's failure to realize until on the verge of suicide that his mother's unmourned death was a central feature of his melancholia suggests that this denial of her importance was a feature too of his superego. The reader is at first invited to judge him harshly for his treatment of his patroness – at this point neither she nor the reader knows about, or can make allowance for, the childhood loss that underlies his behaviour. The patroness and the reader 'actualize' the harsh superego that doesn't know or yet recognize the loss that caused his churlishness. Once the mother's loss and meaning are reinstated, the reader, representing the superego, need judge him neither as mad (biochemically disturbed) nor bad (morally reprehensible). A superego that dismissed the importance of his mother's death may also have rendered Styron unable properly to register what the psychiatric literature told him about maternal loss. Dr Gold, his psychiatrist, would have been an exceptionally poor psychotherapist not to have paid attention to how his depressed patient had handled his mother's death. Styron's superego could not until later allow her loss to matter and thus to render his behaviour intelligible and forgivable to himself.

Because of the darkness visible, the hell that his inner world has become, Styron can find no pleasure or comfort in the world about him. No good or helpful object survives within him and he clings to his wife, a good object in the external world, as if he were a four-year-old child. Where there is no good object within, there is a desperate dependence on any external good object. There is dependence but not, it seems, concern or guilt. By contrast, Roubicek, though deeply attached to Tomas, did not cling to him and did feel keen concern for his fate. Styron's inner state is so devastated that as he plans his suicide he has no thought for the effect upon his wife.

Styron repeatedly acknowledges the staunchness of his wife, but it is in terms, as he himself says, applicable to the mother of a four-and-a-half-year-old terrified of abandonment: 'not for an instant could I let out of my sight the endlessly patient soul who had become nanny, mummy, comforter, priestess and most important, confidante'. Though she is physically present there is little sense of there being a dialogue between them: Styron is outraged that Dr Gold should be so insensitive as to imagine that he has any sexual interest left. By contrast, Roubicek, even though Ruzena is no longer physically with him, maintains for most of the book a lively dialogue with her in his mind – indeed it is his chief resource. At first he recalls past conversations between them but increasingly in his dreams and his fantasies she makes independent and separate contributions which make his exchanges with her a regenerative intercourse. Because he never completely loses the depressive position and his valuation of the person he has lost, as Styron does, Roubicek remains more capable of the sexual and emotional intercourse which the child needs to allow the parents to have. It is upon the internalization of such creative intercourse that the capacity to think creatively depends. Styron, in his melancholia, loses his capacity to think creatively – instead his mind is tyrannized and paralysed by melancholic 'demons'. Roubicek, despite his isolation and the tyranny of the Nazis, is able to sustain a constructive psychic intercourse with the woman he loves: he can think sanely about the cruel and horrific world in which he has to live.

Styron searches for help but to no avail. The psychiatrist he consults under-estimates his suicidal state and gives him inappropriate medication which makes his condition worse. Though in reality far better placed than Roubicek was to find a helpful object, he goes instead to Dr Gold, who makes these serious errors. Anger and resentment may have unconsciously contributed to Styron's choosing a psychiatrist he could later blame and dismiss as incompetent. Competent psychiatrists in New England must be more plentiful and accessible than members of the Czech resistance prepared to shelter Jews in Nazi Prague. The state of our two protagonists' internal objects, and of their relationship to them, affects their judgment and their capacity to find and use help.

He describes a state of 'anxiety, agitation and unfocussed dread'. The dread did to some extent focus on his body, producing a 'pervasive hypochondria'. He suggests that the mind prefers to re-locate its own sense of disaster into the body. A Kleinian view is that the bodily organs may represent unconsciously the phantasied state of the internal objects – deteriorating, neglected and threatening. The state of his internal objects was projected on to his external environment.

> One of the unforgettable features of this stage of my disorder was the way in which my own farmhouse, my beloved home for 30 years, took on for me at that point when my spirits regularly sank to their nadir, an almost palpable quality of ominousness ... I wondered how this friendly place, teeming with such memories of ... 'Lads and Girls,' of 'Laughter and ability and Sighing/And Frocks and Curls' could almost perceptibly seem so hostile and forbidding.

In the internal world 'my beloved home' represents the good internal mother 'teeming' with life and children offering comfort and restoration. He perceives this internal home now as ominous, 'hostile and forbidding'. He feels his objects persecute him and threaten him with annihilation.

At the root of his melancholia lies this dismissal of the importance of his mother and of her loss. Like his French hostess's lunch and the money she gave him, it is dismissed, and, as the story unfolds, in danger of becoming irretrievable.

That her dismissed, unmourned loss is central to his melancholic condition is made clear by the manner of his recovery. As he prepares to kill himself, he chances to hear on the radio a woman singing Brahms' Alto Rhapsody, a song his mother used to sing. He is deeply moved and he recovers his wish to live. The family home revives in his mind as a loved place in which children were reared – a maternal space for growing children that once more is alive with meaning. He recovers his absent good object within him and can then energetically mobilize his wife to save his life by getting him into hospital. He has re-found the equivalent of Roubicek's Materna, an object that will take him to a safe place and protect him from the annihilation that threatens him within.

Styron, as he recovered, came to recognize the part played in his illness by 'incomplete mourning' for his mother and how he had carried within himself 'an insufferable burden of which rage and guilt, and not only damned up sorrow, are a part, and become the potential seeds of self destruction'. After his illness, in considering the effect on him of hearing the Brahms Alto Rhapsody, he recalls that his mother had at that time been 'much on my mind'. Did the music complete an unconscious struggle between the anger and guilt, expressed in his behaviour towards his French hostess (a nullification of what his original maternal object had offered him) and on the other hand a capacity to recover his good objects and his concern for them?

> In a flood of swift recollection [on hearing the music] I thought of all the joys the house had known: the children who had rushed through its rooms, the festivals, the love and work, the voices and the nimble commotion, the perennial tribe of cats and dogs and birds ... All this I realized was more than I could ever abandon, even as what I had set out so deliberately to do was more than I could inflict on those memories and upon those, so close to me, with whom those memories were bound.

The severe melancholic has lost his good internal object and is at the mercy of forces which threaten him with annihilation. He has regressed into the paranoid-schizoid position. While ill, Styron seems to have felt no concern for his wife and no sense that the violence of his state and of his suicidal intentions would 'inflict' suffering on her. It is with the recovery of loving, missing feelings towards his long-dead mother that his objects, internal and external, recover their value. In response he knows he wishes to save them from what, through his suicide he had planned to 'inflict' on them. He recovers himself to protect and repair them.

The recovery of his mother's significance saves Styron's sanity as Roubicek's internal communion with Ruzena saves his. The disparaging dismissal of good objects begins however to reassert itself during Styron's stay in hospital – the efforts of his various therapists are mocked. The art therapist may think she contributed to his recovery but he makes it plain he thinks this is absurd. Is the melancholic cycle resuming with a renewed attack upon external objects which will then be introjected as worthless and/or retaliatory?

Roubicek is able to sustain his sense of a loved and life-giving internal object – his knowledge that the stars belong to him – that he has indeed Life with a Star – and Styron ends his account with the same imagery, quoting Dante, 'And so we came forth and once again behold the stars.'

CHAPTER 5

Beyond the depressive position: Ps(n+1)

RONALD BRITTON

Introduction

When Bion took Melanie Klein's concept of projective identification and extended it to produce his *theory of containment*, he introduced the idea of normal projective identification as part of development, and distinguished this from pathological projective identification. The concept of *containment* both as an important part of infantile development and as a clinical phenomenon is now a well established central tenet of post-Kleinian thinking (see Chapter 12). However, the fact that Bion did something similar in relation to Klein's theory of the paranoid-schizoid and depressive positions has not been so clearly recognized or integrated into Kleinian theory.

Initially, the depressive position was described by Melanie Klein as the underlying psychological state to be found in melancholia. Subsequently, she came to see it as a phase of normal infantile development preceded by what later she called the 'paranoid-schizoid' position. By the time Bion was involved in psychoanalytic theorizing, these two positions were regarded as recurrent throughout life as object-relational complexes or self 'positions' in relation to internal and external objects; the paranoid-schizoid position, characterized by splitting, part objects and projection; the depressive position characterized by integration, whole objects and introjection (see Chapters 3 and 4). If we look closely at Melanie Klein's writings we find that she described the paranoid-schizoid position sometimes as a defence against the depressive position, sometimes as a regression from it and sometimes as that part of development preceding it.

Bion adopted and developed the positions suggesting that they alternated in the process of psychic growth and development throughout life. He used the notation familiar in chemistry for dynamic equilibrium to represent this, Ps←→D. If we follow the implications of Bion's alternating Ps←→D and equate Ps and D with these two positions, then movement *from* the depressive position *to* the paranoid-schizoid position *as well as the other way round* is to be seen as part of a normal process of development. He was concerned to distinguish his *Ps* state from the *pathological* paranoid-schizoid position that Melanie Klein had described. He wrote that where material emerges related to things unknown, 'Any attempt to cling to what [is known] must be resisted for the sake of achieving a state of mind analogous to the paranoid-schizoid position.' He was emphatic that this *Ps* state should be tolerated, 'until a pattern "evolves"'. This 'evolved state' he called *D*, 'the analogue to the depressive position'. He added, 'the passage from one to the other may be very short, ... or it may be long' (Bion, 1970, p. 124). To this end he suggested calling Ps '*patience*' and D '*security*': neither of these terms has caught on.

In this chapter I describe a model which makes the distinction between developmental and pathological movement (Britton, 1998a). It is based on a modification of Bion's formula and makes use of John Steiner's concept of pathological organizations (Steiner, 1987). In this model the movement from paranoid-schizoid to depressive to paranoid-schizoid position (Ps→D→Ps) is seen as part of a continuous, life-long, cycle of development. The term *regression* is limited to describe a retreat to *a pathological organization* which might resemble either D or Ps. This differs from its customary usage.

Regression has usually been taken by Kleinians to mean a backwards movement from the depressive position to the paranoid-schizoid position but in recent times Kleinian writers have rarely used the word. If we were to describe a move *from* a depressive position, with its sense of psychic order, to a paranoid-schizoid position, with its quality of disorder, *as regressive* then Bion's D→Ps could be seen as a form of *regression necessary for development.* This would mean it had something in common with the ideas put forward by several authors that there was a kind of regression in analysis that was helpful. Kris's concept of *regression in the service of the ego* (1935) was probably the first of these. Balint's *regression for the sake of recognition* seems to be a similar notion (1968) and Rosenfeld's '*partial acting out*' as a '*necessary part of any analysis*' has some resemblance to it (1964). Winnicott in the 1950s and '60s was probably the analyst who emphasized most the therapeutic use of what he called *organized regression.* When he first introduced it there were contentious discussions on analytic technique taking place which made it a complex and controversial issue. It has remained so, emerging, rather like Ferenczi's 'active technique' (Ferenczi and Rank, 1924), from time to time with renewed controversy. I suspect the different uses and associations of the term have led to *regression* being dropped from the clinical vocabulary of many psychoanalysts. Therefore before using it in this model I need to discuss the history of the concept of regression and to make clear my use of the term.

Regression

Freud took the view that every mental illness involves some degree and some form of regression to early fixation points. He distinguished between topographical, temporal and formal regression. In other words he saw regression as a return to an earlier pattern of object relating; to more primitive emotional expression and to a style of mentation closer to perceiving than thinking (Freud, 1900, SE 5, p. 548).

In 1943 as part of the *Controversial Discussions* Susan Isaacs and Paula Heimann wrote a paper on the changes in the theory of regression in the light of Melanie Klein's work (Heimann and Isaacs, 1952). They pointed out that parallel with the regression of libido was the regression of the destructive instinct which was more significant in producing psychopathology; this made regression seem more dangerous and less benign. In 1946 the concept of the paranoid-schizoid position was launched by Melanie Klein and formed together with the depressive position what was then seen as 'a coherent and comprehensive theory of psychological development and its pathology' (Segal, 1979, p. 125). From this point onwards regression was usually taken by Kleinians to mean a backwards movement from the depressive position to the paranoid-schizoid position. The words regression and fixation continued to be part of Melanie Klein's personal psychoanalytic vocabulary and that of Herbert Rosenfeld, but other Kleinian writers have hardly used either word. Betty Joseph, in a rare use of the term, wrote 'we see a patient ... better able to face depressive pain, now temporarily regressing in the face of anxieties about the past holiday and particularly the planning of terminating analysis. *She regresses to an earlier defensive system* [my italics], using mechanisms belonging more to the paranoid-schizoid position, splitting, projective identification, and so on' (Joseph, 1989, p. 125). I would ask you to note that Betty Joseph describes the patient as *regressing to an earlier defensive system* and *not to an earlier phase* and she adds that this defensive system uses mechanisms belonging more to the paranoid-schizoid. In this passage she uses another concept commonplace in Kleinian thinking by this time, namely that of '*the defensive system*', first introduced by Joan Riviere (1936). It is clear that Betty Joseph in this passage equates regression with a retreat from the depressive position to a defensive system using mechanisms characteristic of the paranoid-schizoid position. This is usually what is implied by the term *regression* in Kleinian writing since 1952.

Meanwhile, as I mentioned earlier, others such as Winnicott and Balint had been speaking of the desirability of regression in analysis. However, whereas Winnicott wrote positively of protracted and extensive regression, Balint warned against a kind of wholesale regression that was malignant (Balint, 1968, p. 141). Bion, like most other Kleinians after 1952, did not use the term *regression* in his writings. However, in 1960, when the subject of *organized regression* in analysis was a contentious subject in the British Society, he wrote in his notebook, 'Winnicott says patients *need* to regress: Melanie Klein says they *must not*: I say they *are* regressed' (Bion, 1992, p. 166).

I do not want to enter into that debate in this chapter but I would like to emphasize a distinction Winnicott made in his paper on 'Metapsychological and clinical aspects of regression' in which he advocated *organized regression*. He wrote 'an organized regression is sometimes confused with pathological withdrawal and defensive splittings of various kinds. These states are related to regression in the sense that they are defensive organizations.' In contrast to this pathological withdrawal into a defensive organization he refers to a kind of regression that provides a 'new opportunity for an unfreezing of the frozen situation' (1954, p. 283). As I would see it the 'frozen situation' would be a pathological organization and therefore the patient in it is already regressed, as Bion commented.

In order to escape from the language trap of describing good regression and bad regression, I want to reserve the term for a retreat into a pathological organization that reiterates the past and evades the future. I prefer not to use the word regression to describe any developmental move from such a situation towards new opportunities, even though it involves more obvious disturbance and dependence. Often in analysis this apparent regression is the result of hitherto excluded or repressed psychic material which necessarily leads to the loss of the previously achieved psychic organization, and loss of cohesive functioning. This is distinctly different from the regression that takes place in a negative therapeutic reaction for example. The problem, however, remains of distinguishing clinically between a positive psychic development producing turmoil and a pathological regression which reverses development. Pathological regression even in a restricted sense is often benign and short-lived. Like sunburn and the common cold it is however no less pathological for being commonplace and superficial. Pathological regression may be a short-lived hiccough in analysis, or it may be severe and recurrent as in some negative therapeutic reactions, or it may be chronic and disabling resulting in psychiatric disorder.

The 'regression' from the depressive position into a paranoid-schizoid mode of function was first described by Klein and is very familiar in the literature. In my model the resulting paranoid-schizoid pathological organization is referred to as *Ps(path)* to distinguish it from the paranoid-schizoid position of normal development, Ps.

What I most want to emphasize is that in this model the movement from a depressive into *a post-depressive* paranoid-schizoid position, Ps(n+1), is part of normal development: from a coherent belief to incoherence and uncertainty. Regression, when it occurs from this normal *post-depressive* paranoid-schizoid position, Ps(n+1), is into a pathological organization, *a*

quasi-depressive position of certainty which I call *D(path)* ('n' is a mathematical sign denoting the unknown number of Ps to D sequences leading to
the present moment; a low number for 'n' would indicate someone very
young, mentally defective or emotionally immature). There is always a degree
of omniscience in D(path). Similarly when regression occurs from a normal
depressive position, Dn, it is not into a *normal* pre-depressive paranoid-
schizoid position but into a pathological organization with paranoid characteristics called Ps(path), also characterized by omniscience.

What also needs to be emphasized, because it is not familiar, is the regression from a *post-depressive* paranoid-schizoid position [Ps(n+1)] into a defensive organization in the mode of the depressive position, [D(path)]. That is
from a current, emergent state of uncertainty, and incoherence, Ps(n+1), to a
ready made, previously espoused, coherent, belief system [D(path)]. A move
that is prompted by a wish to end uncertainty and the fears associated with
fragmentation. D(path) resembles the depressive position in its coherence,
its self-cognizant mode and its moral rectitude. But it is without the anguish,
humility, resignation and sadness of the depressive position; the place of guilt
and remorse familiar in the depressive position may be taken by masochistic
suffering at the hands of an internal moral supremacist. What characterizes
D(path) is its underlying, omniscient, belief system. The mood associated
with this might be manic or it might be melancholic: if the self is identified as
the omniscient, moral supremacist then it is manic; if the self is the object of
the moral supremacist's flagellations then it is melancholic. In either case
dogmatic certitude is the mode.

Towards a model of psychic development and regression

The normal paranoid-schizoid position is referred to as the *pre-depressive
position* [Ps(n)] when it precedes D(n) and as the *post-depressive position*
[Ps(n+1)] when it follows D(n). The critical *clinical* difference is that in the
pre-depressive position the crisis is the approach of the depressive position,
whilst in the *post-depressive position* the crisis is the loss of cognitive and
moral confidence and the resultant incoherence and uncertainty. It is this
second crisis, that of the *post-depressive position*, which leads to refuge in a
pathological organization that offers coherence on a basis of dogma or
delusion, D(path).

The normal depressive position as described by Melanie Klein and
explored and developed by Hanna Segal is a rich mine of clinical understanding. It encompasses developments in object relations, in the relationship to reality, in the capacity to make distinctions between internal and
external, and it describes crucial developments in the cognitive and moral

spheres. It is not surprising then that arriving at and working through the depressive position should be seen as a psychic achievement and should often be taken to be the aim of analysis and quite possibly of life itself. The elucidation of the development inherent in the move from paranoid-schizoid morality to depressive position thinking, from Talion law to reparation through love, has given the depressive position moral value. In addition Hanna Segal has shown how the move from the paranoid-schizoid to the depressive position makes symbolic thinking possible which gives it reparative power and aesthetic value (Segal, 1952, 1957; see also Chapter 10).

Nevertheless, the Kleinian theory of cognition as it has developed from the 1960s onwards implies that the depressive position is not a final resting place: that leaving the security of depressive position coherence for a new round of fragmented persecuting uncertainties is necessary for development. The only alternative to continuous development *is regression*; that in a world of flux an attempt to stand still produces a retreat: yesterday's depressive position becomes tomorrow's defensive organization.

Reluctance to lose moral sensibility and apparent sanity adds to the problem of relinquishing the depressive position. Once $D(n)$ is relinquished triangular space and therefore reflective thinking is lost and only regained in a new depressive position, the form of which is not only unknown but unimaginable at this point. In $Ps(n+1)$ the ability is gone to put ideas in perspective, to see round things rather than being immersed within them or inhabited by them. Such is the onward movement within an analysis; from integration to disintegration to be followed by re-integration.

In order to clarify the model I will start by putting Klein's theory of the two positions into Ps and D nomenclature.

Klein's theory of the psychic positions expressed as Ps and D

In the beginning there is the infantile paranoid-schizoid position which in time evolves into the infantile depressive position. This process can be represented as $Ps(1) \rightarrow D(1)$. Klein made it clear that they also represented characteristic psychic states and modes of object relating that recur repeatedly throughout life in whatever is the psychic currency of the day. The *present version* is designated as $Ps(n) \rightarrow D(n)$; the version destined to take place some time in the future as $Ps(n+1) \rightarrow D(n+1)$ (see opposite).

As noted earlier 'n' is a mathematical sign denoting the unknown number of $Ps \rightarrow D$ sequences leading to the present moment. Were it knowable, a low number for 'n' would indicate either someone very young, mentally defective or emotionally immature.

$$[Ps(1) \rightarrow D(1) \rightarrow] \qquad \rightarrow Ps(n) \rightarrow D(n) \rightarrow \qquad [Ps(n+1) \rightarrow D(n+1)]$$

Past   Present   Future

Figure 5.1

In Klein's model the progressive movement is from Ps to D in each new situation, and further Ps and D positions lie waiting in the future to be realized in the individuals' object relationships of their day.

Bion's model Ps←→D

Bion proposed that thinking arises to deal with thoughts; thoughts require containing, naming and integrating. He saw D as producing a shape, and the process of *containment* as giving this shape meaning. For this to occur it was necessary to remain in the Ps position long enough for the *selected fact* to emerge which would configure the other fragmented facts by their relationship to it. This crystallization leads to a coherent pattern of thought which he called D. He expressed the oscillation between incoherence and coherence as Ps←→D.

I find this notation resembles the familiar chemical formula for dynamic equilibrium with its oscillation between two unchanging substances. This as a psychological analogy suggests 'reversible perspective' more than psychic development and so I prefer to rewrite it as:

$$Ps(n) \rightarrow D(n) \rightarrow Ps(n+1) \rightarrow ....???? D(n+1).$$

The post-depressive paranoid-schizoid position designated Ps(n+1) results from new knowledge or newly emergent, previously segregated psychic material. It is not a point of arrival like the depressive position [D(n)] but of departure. If Ps(n+1) is thought of as 'the wilderness' of the Exodus then the as yet unseen promised land is D(n+1). Ps(n+1) is a psychic development that is necessarily accompanied by some existential anxiety and narcissistic loss. In some it may produce such profound fear of chaos that this may provoke regressive flight from uncertainty. In others, pride in their knowledge and potential envy of those who appear more confident prevents the relinquishment of coherence and certainty and so refuge is sought in the reinvention of the past [D(path)] masquerading as an unchanging present.

Psychic growth through cycles of Ps(n)→D(n)→Ps(n+1) →....????D(n+1)

In this scheme Ps(n), D(n) and Ps(n+1) represent actual states of mind which are encountered in practice. But D(n+1) only represents a future possibility. It exists only as hope resting on faith. In Bion's terms, it is a *preconception* of a future as yet unimaginable integrating *conception*. Once this preconception is realized it will become the D(n) of its day; in the meantime it is like 'the promised land', only an article of faith.

As a new D(n) becomes imaginable, that is conceivable though not yet conceived, Ps(n+1), the post-depressive state, becomes a new pre-depressive position, or Ps(n). Its character changes as a new resolution becomes imaginable; at first evoking alternating expectations of an ideal solution and persecuting disappointment. The crisis is then, once more, integration and the approach to the depressive position, which is so well described and familiar in the literature.

The cycle has moved on a step; D(n+1), a pre-conception has become D(n), a conception. Figure 5.2 is like a *still frame* from a *moving picture*; it is *not* a *still photograph* nor a photograph of still life. In this sense every account of an analysis that describes a particular moment is a freeze frame.

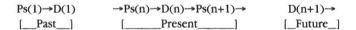

Ps(1)→D(1)	→Ps(n)→D(n)→Ps(n+1)→	D(n+1)→
[__Past__]	[_____Present_____]	[_Future_]

Figure 5.2

Development and regression using the concept of psychic retreats

Following the description in the work of Herbert Rosenfeld and others of a *narcissistic organization* within the personality as offering an alternative to reality and to object-relating, John Steiner produced the concept of *pathological organizations* (Steiner, 1987). He developed this further with his description of them as providing a refuge from reality as *psychic retreats* (Steiner, 1993). It is to such refuges that I see regression taking place. The model I offer below is an attempt to describe in abstract terms the forward movement of psychic development in life and in analysis and the regression into psychic retreats organized either as quasi-paranoid-schizoid positions or quasi-depressive positions.

Figure 5.3 shows *the model of development and regression*. It describes in this scheme of notation the movement that constitutes development from Ps(n) through D(n) and Ps(n+1) towards D(n+1); regression describes the backward move into pathological organizations D(path) or Ps(path).

Development →   Ps(n)   →D(n)   →Ps(n)→D(n)→Ps(n+1)→...............D(n+1)
     ↓   ↓   ↓
←Regression   ←Ps(path)←D(path)
     ↓   ↓   ↓
Recovery→   Ps(n)   →D(n)   →Ps(n+1)→......D(n+1)

Figure 5.3

Figure 5.3 also illustrates the lines of regression and recovery. It is laid out in this way to emphasize that recovery entails the resumption of the developmental line by moving into a new normal paranoid-schizoid or depressive position.

Development and regression in practice

To show these positions and the possible movements between them in practice I will give two brief sketches of different analytic situations. The first is one where the patient moves through analysis with brief episodes of regression and fairly rapid recovery such as one expects in an ordinary analysis. The second is one where severe regression both in terms of extent and duration was always a possibility.

In the first case the brief extract shows these movements on a small scale within the sessions of less than a week of analysis.

1. Cycles of development and regression in ordinary analysis

In the first example the frequently described and familiar movement from structured paranoid defence, through a more fluid paranoid-schizoid position to the depressive position is rapidly traversed. The initial sticking place or point of regression in this analysis appeared to be at the point of development *from* the depressive position into a *post-depressive* position: from integrated understanding into a new situation of uncertainty and incoherence, from D(n)→Ps(n+1).

The patient, a young woman social worker, had left the previous day's session having been quite insightful in a sad reflective mood. She arrived next day five minutes late in an angry mood, feeling persecuted but communicative. 'I don't know why I am late,' she said in an exasperated way.

She then began talking angrily about a new woman colleague with whom she now shares an office in her department. This woman doesn't listen, she said. She had told her not to put her things in that area of the office, which they shared, without agreement. But she went ahead and did so; this made the office unbearable for my patient. 'This woman's things are horrible,' she said, while implying that her own were pleasing and in good order. At some length she complained of the impossibility of her colleague and suspected her disruptiveness might have an ulterior motive. (I would describe my patient's movement overnight as from the depressive position D(n) into a pathological organization organized on paranoid lines Ps(path).)

I commented, 'Where there is a difference in taste and when unfamiliar objects are introduced by someone else, there is a problem not just about physical space but about shared mental space and whose mental space is it.'

'Yes!' said the patient, 'I have to *see* her things! They fill my mind!'

The patient continued to complain that her colleague's alien objects and different ways disrupted the pre-existing pristine harmony of the office. She could not see how such a situation could be solved except by getting rid of her. Her state was now one of persecutory feeling associated with a sense of intrusion and a desire to be rid of something but it was more distressed than suspicious; more fragmentary than organized. [I would describe this as a move to a normal pre-depressive paranoid-schizoid position Ps(n).]

I then linked this situation to the transference. I spoke of the problem of the shared mental space of the analysis and that if I introduced anything new into it without her agreement, and which did not accord with her way of looking at things, it felt to her as though I spoiled her way of seeing things.

There was a short silence then she said 'That's right!' After a longer silence and in a quieter voice the patient said, 'Dr Britton, how am I going to change?' After a short pause she continued, 'You see how I am. It's true, I persecute this poor woman. I'm intolerant, and I don't want to listen to you a lot of the time. It feels hopeless, how can anyone like that ever be the sort of person who can think of helping other people?' [I would describe this as a move into the depressive position D(n).]

I commented, 'You can see the need to change in some ways but you despair of doing so. You are ready to blame yourself for this but I think you do not realize that it also indicates that you have no belief that analysis can do anything for you either.'

(long pause)

Patient: 'That's true ... it is ... I hadn't realized it but when I think about it I don't have any expectation that you will make any difference at all; I do think it's all up to me and that no-one is capable of helping me.'

(pause)

'That is surprising ... I never realized that. How did you know I thought that? I didn't know ... (pause) How does one do that? It never occurred to me; I don't understand really but it's true,' she said, and then paused as if lost in thought.

[I would see this as a move into a post-depressive paranoid-schizoid position, what I have termed Ps(n+1). The persecutory aspect of this advance rapidly became evident in the next shift in the session.]

After a short silence she resumed in a more decisive voice, 'Now I feel so discouraged ... I will never be able to do that! ... I will never learn to do that!'

This then became a springboard for a familiar reaffirmation of inferiority, pessimism about her future, under-valuation of her abilities and an over-valuation of mine, all in an omniscient mode.[(I would regard this as regression to a familiar somewhat masochistic psychic retreat D(path)).]

I said 'Having discovered your lack of belief in me you became anxious about what your scepticism might do to my self-belief so now you are set on restoring it by attributing to me permanent possession of all the abilities you would like to have yourself; this puts you in the miserable but reassuringly familiar position of reproaching yourself for your inferiority whilst idealizing me.'

The patient responded by saying 'I remember now why I was late, I really didn't want to come. I was hating you a great deal before coming today.'

The patient finally ended the session speaking sadly of her mother whose intrusiveness and imperviousness she frequently complained about and had hated as a child. But she now spoke of feeling guilty when she thought of her mother's life-long depression. The patient remained thoughtful, rather sad, but now seemed quietly confident. [I would describe her as in D(n), that is in the depressive position proper at the point at which she left.]

Next day

Coming to a new session having had an insightful dream which faced her with unaccustomed thoughts and hence a move towards Ps(n+1), the patient then regressed. She arrived late for her session, full of self-reproach and absolutely sure she was disliked. She asserted that I was superior in every way and above reproach; she was inferior, stupid and unable to learn. The mood was melancholic; the mental state omniscient. I would describe this as D(path), a quasi-depressive psychic retreat. This retreat was for her an uncomfortable but reassuringly familiar, equilibrated state of mind but for the analyst, frustrating and apparently impermeable. The patient stayed in this position throughout that session and then in the following one moved once again into a normal depressive position. After giving vivid expression to her envious feelings, her impatience, hatred of herself for knowing less and of me for knowing more, she moved into a state of sadness, resignation and guilt. By the end of that session a quiet sense of hope emerged from the depressive position.

Further developments meant that patient and analyst had to confront new uncertainties in the analysis and the need once more to relinquish the coherence of the depressive position for the incoherence of Ps(n+1). This again was to prove too difficult. Thus there were to be further cycles of development and regression which to use another old term, I would call *working through*.

2. More prolonged severe regression

The second passage of analysis to which I want to refer was very different. The patient could be said to belong to that group Rosenfeld described as *thin-skinned narcissistic* patients whom I think of as people given to a *hypersensitive subjectivism*.

The episode is from a long analysis that took place some time ago, so I can speak from a position of hindsight. At the point where my brief account begins, the patient, a man, was in the state of mind I would characterize as the depressive position, D(n). He was, after years of analysis that included much violence and considerable pain, in a state of mind of guilt, regret and sadness. It also included curiosity about me and conscious feelings of love and hate. He then, inadvertently, made a new discovery, namely, the identity of another patient. It was a particularly significant discovery because the fellow patient was in the same field of the fine arts as the patient himself. To add to his provocation his newly discovered analytic sibling was undoubtedly gifted and more publicly established than the patient. The new discovery was like the birth of a new sibling. His reaction exposed the fact that his hard-won acceptance of life, and of his analysis was based on a belief that he was unique among my patients. This resembled his childhood belief about his family position, as the only boy, before the birth of a younger brother. Initially this fragmented his thinking and feelings. It moved him from the depressive position into a new paranoid-schizoid position, or Ps(n+1).

I believe this is always the case. *It is what happens next which really matters.* Is it going to be possible to move on to a new, as yet unimaginable, resolution incorporating the new facts in what I have called D(n+1), some depressive position of the future? Or is a regression to a pathological organization likely to take place and if it does, how long is that going to persist? A further possibility was demonstrated in this case when the initial regression to a psychic retreat did not hold and further regression to more primitive pathological organizations took place. I think this is the sort of sequence that Michael Balint meant by *malignant regression*.

To return to the moment in question in this analysis when the patient felt shattered by the new discovery, his previous sense of having a special unique position in relation to the analyst was undone. He was no longer, even in his own mind, the only one. If he was not, then who was he, what was he and where was he in relation to me? In short he was in a new psychic situation with all his previous assumptions in pieces - Ps(n+1). Unable to bear the sense of fragmentation and associated fear of chaos, he rapidly regressed to a pathological organization, D(path). This took a melancholic form: the patient asserted that he knew he was hopeless, someone contemptuously regarded by everyone; not only was he an unacknowledged outcast but he deserved to be. There was no doubt in his mind that I despised him.

Some patients might at this point work their way out of this by relinquishing melancholic omniscience and find their way back from absolute
worthlessness to a more realistic sense of their relative inferiority and the
feelings accompanying that of jealousy and envy; in other words moving
towards a true depressive position. Others might remain in this place D(path)
by sustaining a steady state of moral masochism and develop a chronic
depression. Others might stay in the same moral zone while producing a
manic reversal of roles and become through projective identification, a
superior person contemptuous of all inferiors such as those foolish enough
to admire this new analytic sibling's work.

However, none of these things occurred. Melancholic and manic
positions rapidly alternated but neither was sustained, instead, unable to bear
self-reproach and unable to achieve manic superiority, the patient regressed
into a structured paranoid organization, Ps(path). He was now outraged, and
not simply enraged; he was convinced that he had been exposed to knowledge from which he should have been protected by me as his analyst. It was,
he implied, a conspiracy to humiliate him; first by keeping him ignorant of it
and not preparing him and then allowing him to be exposed to it. It sounds
unconvincing as I say it but it was not at the time when the atmosphere in the
sessions was that of a trial with the analyst and analysis in the dock.

This self-righteous state of chronic grievance which Michael Feldman has
described (1995) as a defensive organization continued for a long time. It was
a means of channelling hatred while the grievance acted as a focus that
functioned as a psychic organizer holding the patient's thinking together. In
this way it provided him with a psychic container protecting him from his
fears of fragmentation.

Whenever he moved out of this judicial mode it was first into a more
generalized persecutory state and then a move towards concern for the
analyst and a reappraisal of himself. This move towards the depressive
position would usually founder when he made an adverse comparison of
himself as an analytic patient with me or with other imaginary patients.
Shame and humiliation would then displace guilt and remorse and the
restoration of pride took precedence over reconciliation which moved him
back into his paranoid organization, Ps(path), for another round of grievance.

The problems in approaching or sustaining the depressive position are
well described and it is not my intention to add to them here or to speculate
on aetiology or psychopathology. I simply wanted to describe the movement
within the framework of this model of a case in analysis where there was a
marked tendency to chronicity.

As I quoted earlier, Bion stated when speaking of the move from Ps to D,
'the passage from one to the other may be very short, as in the terminal stages
of analysis, or it may be long'. In this case the passage was not only very long

but it was also complicated by many regressions, and sometimes compound regressions, into pathological organizations that removed it from the developmental line.

To summarize what has been said in this chapter: I have suggested opening out Bion's formula to read: $Ps(n) \rightarrow D(n) \rightarrow Ps(n+1) \rightarrow ?$ with $D(n+1)$ somewhere over the psychic horizon. In addition to the familiar *pre-depressive* paranoid-schizoid position, which is characterized by the anxiety of integration, a *post-depressive* position has been described characterized by *de-integration* which may lead to fears of disintegration. Although in the *post-depressive* position, $Ps(n+1)$, certain functions associated with the depressive position are temporarily lost, it is not regression but transition. The term regression is reserved in this system to describe a retreat to a pathological organization. This organization might be in the paranoid or depressive mode, Ps(path) or D(path).

The pre-depressive, the depressive and the post-depressive positions are all states of mind we experience in ourselves and meet in clinical practice. Unlike these, $D(n+1)$, which represents a future but as yet unimaginable resolution, is not a state of mind that is ever experienced. It is a hope, based on faith, that future developments will bring coherence and meaning. It is in Bion's terms a pre-conception. To put this in mythic terms, the post-depressive position, $Ps(n+1)$, is 'the wilderness' and $D(n+1)$ is 'the promised land'. By the time it is near to realization $D(n+1)$ has become the familiar depressive position $D(n)$: the promised land has become Israel and another struggle has begun.

The clinical phenomenon I particularly want to draw attention to is the regressive movement that frequently takes place from the post-depressive position of fragmented belief and moral ambiguity to the intellectual coherence and moral certainty of D(path). It is a common journey and in the intellectual sphere it is a path that has felt the tread of some distinguished feet. Even Einstein when faced with the new mathematics of the 'uncertainty principle' refused to believe it, feeling that the Almighty would never have created such a crazy place as the Universe of Quantum Mechanics. 'Strange but true,' said Neil Bohr when faced with it; 'too weird to be credible,' said Einstein (Polkinghorne, 1986, p. 55). Perhaps Freud in his last period also retrenched, no longer saying *strange but true* but instead *too weird to be credible*, when Melanie Klein pushed even further into the hinterland of unconscious phantasy.

CHAPTER 6

The Oedipus Complex

JILL BOSWELL

A patient who had no children dreamed that she was pregnant. 'In the dream I have a big, hard belly, I must be near time,' she said. We discussed the dream, including its possible connection with the five-week summer break in the analysis, which was imminent. For patients in analysis a break can be difficult to bear, as it makes them acutely aware that their analyst has a separate private life. On this occasion something the patient said about her dream led me to comment that this heavily pregnant version of herself sounded uncomfortable and she might be looking forward to the baby being born. She appeared quite struck with this idea; for a long time she had clung to a belief that nothing could be more desirable for a mother and baby than a state of endless pregnancy. This belief was linked with her wish to be part of such a mother-and-baby entity. While admitting it was irrational, she nonetheless believed it would protect her from realities she dreaded, such as the summer break when we would be apart. My comment on her dream seemed to touch a growing awareness in her, which she took up again in the next session.

First, she said she was feeling angry, and thought it was because of the break, saying, 'I've realized it's going to happen.' After a number of complaints and angry remarks her tone altered as she went on to report that she had gone shopping that morning, and noticed behind her in the queue a young woman who was obviously pregnant. The patient told me: 'I asked her, "Would you like to go first – unless you will be a long time?" and the young woman answered, "Sixteen days!"' They both laughed, and the woman explained, 'I can't think of anything else!' My patient added, to me, 'I realized you were right yesterday. Someone who had had a baby would know that.' In spite of her resentment she seemed more able to understand the mother's wish for the baby to be born and by implication, link it to my break. The warmth and humour of her story conveyed that the break was not simply felt

77

as an intolerable rejection of her. In her mind she could give up her omnipotent control over me, representing the mother behind her, and allow me to go first as it were, to have my break, or my baby.

Later she talked about looking for a new job in the autumn, as her present one allowed her no room for her own ideas, and she commented that she felt less desperate about the break this year, although she knew she was still angry with me for leaving her. I interpreted to her that she felt something creative could come from facing the analytic break, although the price to her seemed very high – agreeing to be born so to speak, allowing me my holiday away from her. She acknowledged this, but said again that this year it was only a break, not such a disaster as it had used to seem. After a pause she wondered if there would be any changes to the room when she returned in September.

I said, 'You mean while you are away, and maybe even thinking about your new job, I might have some new ideas of my own, or with my husband, and things might be different when you get back.' I interpreted in this way because I thought my patient was struggling with the idea of a parental couple who, in her mind, would come together while she was absent. One outcome of the parents' relationship, a new pregnancy, would become possible once she had left, and I thought this unconscious thought was behind her reference to changes in my consulting room.

The patient quite angrily retorted that my husband had nothing to do with this room. 'This is your consulting room. I doubt if he knows or cares what happens here.'

I said, 'I brought him in, and you immediately want to push him out.'

She was silent for a moment, but then spoke of a party she had been to over the weekend, where she had met a couple, a woman she thinks I know and her husband, who is in a field related to her own. 'He told me he'd been invited to do some particularly interesting work for my company, and I came out with one of my remarks, you know; I said aggressively, "Why do they ask you?" And his wife said, "Because he is good," which is right. Then I wished I hadn't said that.'

I said, 'I brought in my husband just now, and you said, in effect, "Why him? Why not me?" It made you feel again that I should only want to be in here with you, like a pregnant mother with a baby who is never born. I think you're sorry to be so jealous and aggressive, because you'd like to be more generous. And also, you realize that you yourself would like to be freer to follow your own ideas. But with the break so near you suddenly can't bear me bringing him in, and then you get furious again.'

It was evident that my mentioning my husband had been painfully provocative, and brought an angry response from the patient. She felt acutely the unfairness of having to make way for him even in the consulting room, which I thought represented the mother's body, perhaps the womb. She wanted me to keep it empty until she returned, although she herself had voiced suspicions that changes might occur. The interpretation was intended to help make explicit her thoughts that seemed to be coming to consciousness.

From this clinical interchange it is possible to see that as the more primitive phantasy of an endless mother–baby union starts to lose its grip on her thinking, her thoughts and feelings change in significant ways. First, she is able to feel more separate, and among other things, this enables her to observe – for example, the discomfort of the pregnant woman in the queue. Her considerate gesture, as well as the humour of the story as she told it, suggest that she is now not so dominated by envy and hatred of a couple. Secondly, when hatred and jealousy do erupt in the session, with the thoughts of my husband being invited in to 'her' place during the break, she can express some regret for her attack on him – represented by the husband at the party.

In the predominantly Oedipal themes of these extracts, we can see a patient struggling to express and confront her feelings about the facts of life – about birth, representing both loss and hope, and about the child's exclusion from the parents' sexual relationship with the envy and jealousy that this provokes. Together with the awareness of exclusion goes the experience of finding out, of learning. This process of change and growth always involves pain, but it also opens up the potential for warmer and more generous relationships. Although it was fraught with difficulty for the patient, when she could achieve this shift it did seem to offer her the hope that she too could look forward to a freer relationship not only with her analyst but in her life outside, with the thought that she might find new ways to develop her own creativity.

The working over of such Oedipal conflicts is central to the tasks of an analysis. In Kleinian practice the analyst would watch out for shifts in the patient's thoughts and feelings as they might register movement between the paranoid-schizoid position and the depressive position (see Chapter 5). In the second session I described, the patient was feeling anger towards her analyst, and hatred of the husband, although she did not lose touch with warmer feelings, some guilt, and some concern for the feelings of others. The break, while painful, was not at this point seen as a disaster for her. She was able to observe her objects instead of feeling more or less concretely identified with them, and this was linked with a tolerance of separateness which enabled her also to reflect on her own feelings and also to an extent, think about her future development. The indications seemed to be that she was feeling sufficiently integrated to be able to bear her distress and anger. Although her dream reflected her long-held phantasy of union with the analyst, she could to an extent relinquish it, and though angry she did not seem to feel she was in a hostile world of hatred with no experience of love either given or received.

Such a shift to depressive position functioning can never be complete, and neither can it be permanent (see Chapter 4). In the patient described above, what looked like significant emotional change could be recognized by herself and her analyst, following several weeks of productive work. In subsequent sessions, however, and immediately after the break, she often seemed unable to hold out against more primitive states of mind, which produced hatred of the analyst and of others close to her, and intense anxiety about herself, sometimes experienced as bodily fears of illness and death. These anxieties, more typical of the paranoid-schizoid position (see Chapter 3), were experienced in several contexts: in Oedipal terms they became focused on acute envy and hatred of couples with children.

This raises the question whether the shift towards the depressive position was real or illusory. It might be suggested that the patient was able to talk in the way she did because in these sessions she was, in phantasy, living out the dream in which she herself was pregnant. If the analytic work in the session was unable to disturb a concrete, bodily (though unconscious) belief that she was both mother and baby, then the shift we have noted might have been more apparent than real. Her subsequent failure to maintain it may bear this out. On the other hand, it may have been real enough, but fleeting, not solid enough to withstand the pressures imposed by the coming break and her great difficulty with bearing frustration. Patient analytic work would be needed to discern the long-term trend with more confidence, to enable interpretations to be directed more precisely. In doing this the analyst looks for guidance to the patient's unconscious responses to her, which help with judging the emotional tone and level of the interactions in the session. Later in the chapter we will look at some material from a patient in a more obviously disturbed state of mind, in which primitive mechanisms – phantasies and defences – clearly dominate his thinking.

Melanie Klein and the Oedipus Complex

It was Melanie Klein who first recognized the existence of primitive Oedipal phantasies and wishes, and traced them back to infancy. Her thinking about the Oedipus Complex was grounded on Freud's pioneering work, but she developed the concept in a number of significant ways. Before outlining these we need to look briefly at Freud's concept.

Freud (1905b, 1910b, 1923, 1924) gave the Oedipus Complex a central place in his theory of psychosexual development – a place it continues to hold. By naming his theory for the Greek myth of King Oedipus, who unknowingly killed his own father and married his mother, Freud was drawing attention to the universality of this powerful unconscious complex.

He considered that Oedipal strivings became active in the phallic stage, from three to five years of age, when the penis takes on a special significance for both boys and girls. (The word 'phallic' implies an idea of the symbolic penis, embodying a kind of impregnable power, and is ascribed by children to both parents before they discover anatomical differences.) He recognized both a negative and a positive form of the Oedipus Complex, according to whether the desire of the moment was for the parent of the same sex or the opposite. For the boy child, Freud thought the positive Oedipus Complex involved genital wishes towards the mother, with the attendant jealousy of the father giving rise to murderous feelings against him. The father then became a frighteningly retaliatory figure, forbidding the sexual desires and threatening to castrate the child. The boy's fear of castration forced him to renounce his libidinal desires for his parents, and in the usual course of development he would renounce his mother as a sexual object. The forbidding and punitive father would be introjected to form the nucleus of the superego, which 'perpetuates [the father's] prohibition against incest' (Freud, 1923), but also leads to the formation of conscience and a moral sense. The establishment of the superego, ultimately constructed of imagos of both parents though dominated by that of the father, constituted for Freud the resolution – actually the dissolution – of the Oedipus Complex.

With girls, the process was different: once a girl came to realize she had no penis, she could not fear castration. Instead, her lack of a penis became a central preoccupation (penis envy), causing her to turn away from the mother, now a discredited figure, and to seek a penis from the father and ultimately in her own baby, which unconsciously she would equate with a penis. For her, the Oedipus Complex was never resolved; it was more that she accepted a compromise. Freud thought that girls had a specially long and close pre-Oedipal attachment to the mother, which was ruptured by the bitterness of discovering that a female has no penis. He did not think either boys or girls had knowledge of the vagina until they reached genital maturity at puberty. Until then the phallus was held to be the only sexual organ: in phantasy its possession bestowed omnipotence and its loss would lead to grievous mutilation of the self, or even to death.

Melanie Klein's work on early infantile experience led her to make extensive revisions to this theory. She was careful to point out where she agreed with many of Freud's findings, such as the boy's desire for the mother, with the subsequent hatred of and fear of retaliation from, the father. She too thought children of both sexes had phantasies about their own genitals and those of the parents that coloured their wishes and their fears, and she elabor-ated on these extensively in her clinical papers. She also agreed with him that the superego was constructed in the first instance from internalized parental objects. However she startled many of her contemporaries by dating the onset of the Oedipus Complex at around the end of the first year, far earlier than had Freud. One sign of this, she claimed, was the earlier appearance of guilt feelings, observable in the primitive persecutory fears of very young children.

Secondly, she believed that Freud's superego (at 3–5 years) was really an evolved version of an internal object world that had been built up gradually through a process of projection and introjection from the beginning of life (see Chapter 8). Thirdly, she felt the course taken by an individual's Oedipal development depended crucially on his or her first object relationship - that with the mother. The internalized breast was, she thought, soon joined by the internalized paternal penis as the foundation of the superego in its many facets.[1] From this flowed her fourth main area of difference with Freud: over female sexuality. Klein thought both boys and girls had from the start an unconscious knowledge of both male and female genitals. Further, she found that little girls sensed the existence of their internal sexual organs and their potential to bear children. She thought penis envy in females, though common, was not primary. The central envy of the girl was of her mother's feminine characteristics - her breasts and above all, her ability to bear children given her by the father. Klein's fifth disagreement with Freud concerned his theory of the resolution of the Oedipus Complex. Here, as indicated above, she came to link emotional maturation with what she termed 'working through the depressive position'. By 1945 she had revised her earlier finding (1928) that Oedipal experience arose at the time of maximum sadism in infantile life, stating instead that it arose when more loving feelings started to predominate, bringing depressive guilt, concern and reparative wishes. These influenced and interacted with genital desires towards parents, and also with a growing recognition of external reality - including that of the parental relationship. In time she modified Freud's focus on the sexual 'phases' (oral, anal and genital). Instead she emphasized the concept of 'positions' - complex mental states which in essence defined how all emotional and cognitive experience was organized. The concept of dissolution of the Oedipus Complex fell away, since the positions were not thought of as fixed, but relatively fluid in response to external pressures as well as internal feeling states and impulses.

We will now examine briefly these ideas as they developed in Klein's thinking, and later glance at subsequent development of some of them by her colleagues and followers. Although she referred to the Oedipus Complex

---

[1]Kleinians today have largely abandoned the anatomical part-object language that Klein used; they think more in terms of function - 'feeding' for instance - than of 'the breast' as a structure in the mind; see Spillius, 1988a, p. 5.

throughout her writings, her two central papers on this theme are 'Early stages of the Oedipus complex' (1928) and 'The Oedipus complex in the light of early anxieties' (1945).

The early Oedipus Complex

As we have seen, Klein thought that genital feelings emerged towards the end of the first year of life (see Chapter 1). She found that very little children showed evidence of some innate knowledge, or preconception, of both male and female sexual organs, if only in a very primitive way, and also of something representing sexual intercourse and of the origin of babies within the mother's body. However, she observed that in the beginning these crude ideas could only be interpreted through the child's main modalities of experience, closely linked to the body – namely the oral and the anal or urethral. Therefore she suggested; for a baby of either sex the father's penis might first of all be desired orally, which meant some idea of sucking on it as if it were a breast. If hated, it might in phantasy be bitten and devoured and so taken in, or internalized, as a damaged and retaliatory object. (These phantasies would apply, too, to the mother's breast.) The parental intercourse was conceived of in various ways, which might include mutual feeding or violent assault. The baby's rudimentary notion of how the sexual organs might function, contributed to phantasies of the father's penis as concretely inside the mother. If attacked, this internal penis would become dangerous, which added to anxiety about the mother's body. Particularly terrifying was the image of the 'combined object' which seemed to be composed of the parents' bodies brought together in a confused and distorted way in a continuous sadistic intercourse. (The 'combined object' includes the phantasy of the penis inside the mother. Klein thought that this accounted for ideas of the 'phallic woman' suggested by Freud as evidence that children believed women to possess a penis.)

In her paper 'Early stages of the Oedipus complex' (1928) Klein emphasized the role of sadism and primitive envy. However, as she developed her central concepts of the depressive position (1935) and the paranoid-schizoid position (1946) (see Chapters 3 and 4), her thinking moved away from a view of the infant as dominated by its primitive instincts – specifically, envy associated with the death instinct – to a more object-related view of development, underpinned by the interplay of love and hate. Increasingly she emphasized that love for the good object – the maternal breast – was the essential foundation on which could be built a secure inner world. Klein thought that the frustrations inflicted by the mother, weaning in particular, would cause the child to turn to its father, so that his penis (his masculine creative function) would form the second significant internal object. This helped dilute the intense anxiety associated with the 'bad breast', and offered support to the child overwhelmed with guilt produced by its own hatred.

But since at this time the child was becoming aware of its own genital feelings and connecting them with its dawning awareness of a sexual relationship between its parents, further frustrations, including feelings of envy and jealousy towards either parent or both, would cause repeated experiences of rage and distress. These painful emotions could only be faced and worked through with internal support from good objects (see Chapter 7). Without them, emotional development would be impeded. In particular the child would be unable to establish the depressive position, because the integration of good and bad aspects of the object ultimately implied the bringing together in the mind of the sexual parents in a good intercourse.

Acknowledging the fullest play of feelings, good as well as bad, now came to be seen as a major task of growth and development, and it is an important aim in psychoanalytic treatment. It is held to promote awareness of psychic (that is, internal) as well as external reality. It is related to creativity and to the ability to learn.

Klein found that infants had a burning curiosity from early on about their mother's insides, felt as benign or very dangerous according to the infant's current state of mind. Sexual phantasies, when not suffused with sadism and hence anxiety, were for Klein (as for Freud) an important aspect of curiosity and sexual development, and contributed to a child's identification with the loved and admired sexual parent. But when envy was especially strong, including envy of the Oedipal parents, it would feel driven to get inside the mother, to take control and to appropriate the contents including father's penis. The wish to find out would here be connected with aggression, even violence. In phantasy the child would be intruding into the exciting but dangerous body of the mother, to possess or enviously to attack the contents. Klein called this the 'femininity phase', an identification with the mother arising not so much from a desire for sexual union with her as from a wish to possess her attributes (especially her sexual fertility) – to be her. The expected outcome would be violent retaliation by one or other parent, and therefore this intrusive curiosity would be accompanied by severe guilt – the persecutory guilt characteristic of the paranoid-schizoid position. If not modified, the intense anxiety produced by these phantasies might contribute to later learning difficulties – to intellectual as well as to sexual inhibitions – because unconsciously the child became convinced that it was dangerous to be curious and hence, to learn.

These feminine identifications would normally be brief in the boy, but in the girl they formed the basis for her sense of identity as a female. If her phantasied attack on the mother's insides had been particularly fierce and sustained, the girl's terror of retaliation in kind would leave her with profound anxieties about her own body and in particular about her fertility. In favourable circumstances, the girl could turn to a relationship with the 'good penis' of her father for support and to mitigate the force of these anxieties: this would be crucial for her sexual development. For a boy the counterpart would be the terror of castration at the hands of a punitive father thought of as located within the mother's body. A good paternal object was essential for the boy, to identify with as a sexual male and to support him when frightened by his own rivalrous feelings.

The 'femininity phase' is essentially an early sketching out of Klein's theory of projective identification, (1952a), with its implications of intrusion and control of the object (see Chapter 9). This phantasy of identification with the mother can be assumed in the patient's dream that she was pregnant. For her, it seemed to function as a defence against the envious hatred aroused by the imminent analytic break. As the Oedipal phantasies emerged in the sessions, the envy became focused on the parents as a couple, and on their sexual creativity.

Over time and given a reasonably good environment, the violence and concreteness of these early phantasies would gradually diminish. The child would learn to tolerate separateness, relinquish possession of the mother, and become more able to bear its exclusion from the parents' sexual relationship. For Klein, this ability to let go amounted to a form of restitution – a making good of what in phantasy had been taken or enviously destroyed. Such reparation she saw as flowing from a sense of guilt based on remorse and love for a good object. This was an enormously significant step forward from Freud's early concept of the resolution of the Oedipus Complex as founded on the terror of retaliation. For her, the working through of Oedipal conflicts required a capacity for depressive (not persecutory) guilt and concern for the objects – and for these it depended on a superego that was essentially loving and supportive. At the same time, she took care to distinguish between a 'good' and an 'idealized' object, since the facing of reality whether internal or external, necessarily implied a recognition and tolerance of failure and imperfection.

For some, the development of a reality sense may not be reliably achieved. The following clinical description suggests how even in adulthood, primitive phantasies can dominate and distort thinking and perception.

Clinical illustration

A very isolated man had come to analysis because he felt unable to maintain close relationships of any kind. He lived with his parents but kept mainly to his room, where he had become so absorbed in his phantasies that he had difficulty distinguishing between them and reality. On the weekend before the sessions to be discussed he had, very exceptionally, been to an office party. Here he had introduced a young woman he knew slightly, to a male colleague who was single. He at once started to imagine that they had struck up a sexual relationship, brought about by himself.

In his Monday session he described how he had gone home after the party and became obsessed with sexual thoughts about the woman. In the end he had felt forced to masturbate to deal with the excitement. (He often tried to avoid masturbating because the phantasies that accompanied it were disturbingly violent and perverse.) However, he continued to feel very excited and disturbed all weekend. This could be understood as a phantasy of creating and then intruding on, a sexual encounter between a couple representing the parents. It will be noticed that the patient did not imagine himself as excluded from this imaginary relationship, and observing it – he immediately believed he was involved. The feelings this aroused were omnipotent, sadistic and very agitated. Unable himself to approach a woman, he instead felt he had brought the couple together, but then proceeded to eliminate the man and possess the woman.

Immediately after leaving the session in which he recounted this, the patient returned to my house and explained he thought he had left his briefcase in the waiting room. Needing to attend to something before the next patient, I left him in the hall to look for it; he could be heard leaving the house a moment later. The next day he was still in a disturbed state. First, he apologized and said he had not after all left his case here, it had been in the boot of his car all along. Then he told how he had gone to work and his (female) boss had met him and said 'Hello, what's happening with you?' The patient thought she must have heard about the party – and in a delusional way he felt she knew about his masturbation and his intrusive phantasies. He was upset and couldn't answer her; and felt she shouldn't be making use of what she had heard in this way.

I said that he knew that I'd seen him come back yesterday after the session, and he felt I must want to know what he was up to. He was afraid I was suspicious and hostile towards him because I knew all about his thoughts and phantasies about coming in here like that.

He said that in fact he'd been relieved at the time that I didn't seem to mind his coming in. But he had expected me to return to see him out again. In fact he had seen that the door of my consulting room was open, and he could look in. He'd thought he could go in and steal something, and I wouldn't know. He said this with great anxiety.

He told me that later in the day he had gone to the canteen at work, where he drank some coffee and thought about the woman at the party. Now he found himself thinking that I should stop him doing that. His mind then went to another recent incident when he felt he had talked too intimately with a woman who worked with a man senior to himself in the organization. He felt very worried about these things he was doing.

I interpreted that he was very worried that I'd allowed him to come in to this part of my house when I wasn't there – that I should have stopped him doing that, getting in where he wasn't supposed to be – and where he could steal my things – that I should have prevented that from happening. He was now feeling very disturbed, excited and anxious about all these things that seemed to bring him such trouble.

This patient appeared to be in the grip of primitive phantasies about intruding and appropriating first, the parental intercourse, and then, the contents of the mother's body, seen as the consulting room. Possibly he believed unconsciously that his briefcase was a penis, his own or even his father's, left inside me, which he felt compelled to retrieve; but in doing so he became caught up in a further enactment of his phantasy. My failure to stay and see him out had left him in a dangerously excited and anxious state about his own intentions and he became very afraid of being punished. He felt he needed a figure, probably a father, to observe his state of mind and to prevent him doing something destructive. This would be a firm but benign Oedipal figure, able to understand his intense urge to get inside and his envious hatred, but in a non-retaliatory way. Instead of this, he felt he was faced by an accusing figure asking him 'What's happening with you?' which he inter-preted as hostile. The paranoia evident in his reaction to that question was intensified by his conviction that his boss knew what he had been thinking and doing on his own during the weekend – that is, his secret phantasies and activities. This was a counterpart to his own intrusiveness, in which he really seemed to feel he had got inside me; similarly this other figure knew and saw everything, rather as a fearful believer might feel that the eye of God was on him wherever he was.

What this material is intended to illustrate is how the state of a patient's internalized parental objects – his superego – can affect his perception of the world. This patient was in the grip of intense sexualized excitement about being at the party, a rare event for him as his sexual life was at that time entirely a matter of phantasy and masturbation. Real sexual contact was too frightening to him, probably because his violent phantasies made it seem so very dangerous. His involvement in what at once became for him an actual sexual intercourse between the couple at the party, was continued in his mind over the weekend with the phantasies about the woman. His excited intrusion into the scene was then partially enacted with his analyst on the Monday.

Everything that happened was interpreted by the patient in the light of his delusional state. In particular, his internal objects and his relationship to them were projected into external figures, whose ordinary characteristics were significantly changed for him. This could be seen from the encounter later in the day, with his boss: she was usually seen as a friendly and kind figure, but now her casual enquiry carried sinister and hostile overtones. He felt he was able to maintain me as a benign figure (in that I hadn't seemed upset by his return after the session), but the next parent-figure he encountered became unfriendly and punitive.

Depressive feelings mingled with violent and paranoid ideas in this man, and he felt oppressed by his compulsion to masturbate with phantasies of attacking and degrading women. His ability to function sexually with a woman was severely inhibited, probably because his envy and hatred of women led him to feel surrounded by punitive superego figures, both externally and internally. These seemed to be composed of unrealistic part-objects; fragmented aspects of internal objects, damaged by the patient's phantasy attacks and therefore terrifying. The terror might flow from their imagined retaliation, as well as from the distorted, sadistic relationships between them, in his mind. Various fragmented characteristics were then projected on to the people he actually encountered. In the analysis he often spoke of his bitter resentment towards his mother for her neglect of him as a small boy, and he usually expressed this in outbreaks of rage and misery before any analytic break. The longing for a strong, supportive father was a more depressive feature in this patient, and may have reflected his experience of his father as affectionate but weak.

The early relationship to the breast

In Kleinian theory the superego is considered to be built up gradually from the beginning of life, and at first the qualities of internal objects are changeable and fluid, as the interplay of projections and introjections reflect the fragmented phantasies and feeling states of the child. In the early months, or whenever paranoid-schizoid functioning is dominant, it is thought the qualities of the objects are experienced as totally one thing or the other, as a result of splitting carried out to defend the ego from being overwhelmed. This splitting plays a significant role in the child's early attempts to deal with intense feelings about the parents. It is common for one parent to be idealized and the other hated, and these splits, if relatively fluid, may help to preserve a sense of goodness at times of acute jealousy or other stress. However, if a child's loving feelings for, say, its father, are strongly influenced by bitterness and hatred towards its mother, the relationship is likely to be brittle and precarious. Similarly, an idealization of the breast may be established by means of a split which maintains an image of the father as a bad object. If prolonged, this splitting provides a form of retreat to a pre-Oedipal relation to the parents, to defend against intolerable anxiety. In time it is likely to result in an inhibition of the child's own sexual development.

Curiosity, learning, symbolizing

As noted earlier, Melanie Klein regarded curiosity as a central driving force in emotional and cognitive development, and linked it with the earliest stage of the Oedipus Complex. For the child to start freeing itself from the early confused involvement with the mother and her body, a balance of curiosity and anxiety was crucial. A measure of anxiety impelled the child to seek other, less danger-fraught relationships; where this anxiety was not excessive, it would interact with curiosity to stimulate the pursuit of new experience and new objects. Klein herself developed these ideas in her work on symbol-formation (1930), and since then a number of other Kleinian writers have made significant contributions. The connection between symbolization, the task of separating from the primary object, and the depressive position, was further studied by Hanna Segal (1981; see also Chapter 10). Wilfred Bion drew on Freud's work, notably 'Formulations on the two principles of mental functioning' (1911a), and showed in *Learning from Experience* (1962a) and other writings how thinking and learning depended vitally on an attitude to reality that sprang from the earliest relationship to the breast. He used the symbol 'K' – the wish to 'get to know' – to define a fundamental link between two people, giving it equal status with 'Love' and 'Hate'. The obverse of epistemophilia, the wish not to see, Klein called 'scotomization'. John Steiner has examined Sophocles' *Oedipus Rex* in relation to the wish to know and the fear of knowing, in the play's main characters (1985).

Ronald Britton (1989) has explored some connections between a child's acknowledgement of its parents' sexual relationship, and its ability to face reality in a wider sense. Picturing the child at one point of the Oedipal 'triangle', Britton describes the link with each parent as forming two sides of the triangle. The all-important third side is the line joining the two parents to each other, and in recognizing this third link the child is in effect observing the parents in a relationship that excludes itself. The result is 'the closure of the Oedipal triangle by the recognition of the link joining the parents'. Symbolically this creates a mental structure on which is based the capacity to adapt to reality that Melanie Klein associated with facing the Oedipal situation. Here facing reality implies relinquishing omnipotent control of the parents, an essential element in achieving and working through the depressive position. Britton stresses the capacity for objectivity – to position oneself in relation to others, to tolerate observing and being observed, and importantly, to observe oneself. On it depends the ability to integrate observation and experience.

Literary illustration

Some of these ideas are strikingly brought to life in a short novel by Henry James, *The Aspern Papers* (1888), which also offers a compelling illustration of obsessive curiosity. It tells of a literary scholar who has devoted himself to researching the life of a famous poet, now dead, called Jeffrey Aspern. The scholar, never named, seems in a sense to live more in and through Aspern's life and identity than his own. The story is set in Venice, where he has settled for the summer, determined to get access to Miss Juliana Bordereau, an ancient and reclusive lady once the lover of his hero. He believes she still has letters and other documents recording their relationship. He therefore insinuates himself into her household, and finds her living in poverty in a grand but bare palazzo with her ageing niece, a dowdy, downtrodden figure who receives him timidly and explains that they never see anyone and never go anywhere.

In his campaign to get possession of the papers, the narrator perceives that the niece, Miss Tina, could be useful to him. The aunt is suspicious, being secretive and possessive of her relationship with Aspern. However, when she finds the narrator is willing to pay an exorbitant rental she agrees to let rooms to him for the summer. His cynical exploitation of Miss Tina's growing infatuation with him is soon apparent to the reader, but for the narrator the only significant sexual relationship lies in the past. He confides to Miss Tina his desire to lay hands on the letters, and his excitement and anxiety reach a feverish pitch as the old lady seems to be nearing her death. His dread is that, guessing his secret intentions, she may burn the papers before she dies.

In a dramatic scene the narrator steals into the old lady's sitting-room believing her to be on her deathbed, and starts looking around for the papers. James shows us his childishly self-serving attempt to convince himself that Miss Tina really wants him to look into the desk.

> If she didn't so wish me, if she wished me to keep away, why hadn't she locked the door of communication between the sitting-room and the sala? ... she meant me to come for a purpose – a purpose now represented by the super-subtle inference that to oblige me she had unlocked the secretary. ... I didn't propose to do anything, not even – not in the least – to let down the lid; I only wanted to test my theory, to see if the cover *would* move.

We never learn if he was right, because suddenly he turns round.

> Juliana stood there in her night-dress, by the doorway of her room, watching me; her hands were raised, she had lifted the ever-lasting curtain that covered half her face, and for the first, the last, the only time I beheld her extraordinary eyes. They glared at me; they were like the sudden drench, for a caught burglar, of a flood of gaslight; they made me horribly ashamed.

She hisses at him, 'Ah, you publishing scoundrel!'

The emphasis on the old lady's eyes – veiled until this moment – conveys their terrifying glare, both accusing and penetrating. With her eyes she not only accuses him, she exposes him: till that moment he has been able to make himself believe that he is not really doing wrong: 'I only wanted to test my theory', 'not even, not in the least' to open the desk and take the papers. Juliana knows exactly what he is after, and her seeing and knowing suddenly make him 'horribly ashamed'.

When the intruder in the story tries to convince himself that Miss Tina must have meant him to creep in and steal the papers, his thinking seems similar to that of the male patient described earlier, when he thought that by leaving him alone near the open door of my consulting room, I was almost inviting him to go in and 'steal' my things. Interestingly, in both cases this is followed by the appearance of the all-seeing eye. In the patient's case it was his boss asking 'What's happening with you?' so that he thought she must know about his weekend and his thoughts. In *The Aspern Papers* it is Juliana's 'extraordinary' accusing eyes. In Britton's terms, the narrator is observed in the act of prying: he suddenly acquires self-consciousness and sees himself for what he is. For the first time he feels guilt.

In James' story, the narrator is so utterly intent on possessing the papers that he is oblivious to the disturbance and distress he causes, especially to the susceptibilities of the niece. The irony is that all the time the old lady has been planning to make use of his obsession. She wants to draw him into a marriage with Miss Tina which will provide for her after her own death. She leaves her 'Aspern papers' to him in her will, on condition he agrees to the marriage. When the narrator realizes this he flees, and we may feel this is not simply because Miss Tina is dowdy and unattractive. A man more established in his genital sexuality would have seen the impending sexual situation and either avoided it or used it more astutely. His Oedipal curiosity seems, above all, to have been driven by a primitive urge to intrude and to appropriate by getting inside the (symbolically parental) relationship. In the end, Juliana defeats him because her understanding of people and her ability to observe are both more developed than his: for all his cunning and his researching, he knows so little, and for all her reclusiveness and poverty, she knows something more. The reader feels that however briefly, she once had a life and a passionate relationship: the narrator has merely tried to live off other people's passions.

Conclusion

In this chapter we have discussed the pathbreaking work of Melanie Klein on the Oedipus Complex, pointing out how she built on Freud's work while developing and integrating it with important concepts of her own. The relationship between the Oedipus Complex and the depressive position has been emphasized, together with its important link with thinking, learning and acknowledging reality: these ideas in particular have been further explored by later Kleinian writers. Psychoanalytic theory suggests that the act of sexual intercourse is a prototype of all creativity, involving as it does the coming together of two people who in their complementary functions, female and male, are able to give life to a third. The painful and difficult task of relinquishing the phantasy of sexual possession of the parents is seen as an essential factor in emotional and intellectual development. Though never completed, the struggle is central to creativity and the work of reparation in the inner world.

CHAPTER 7

Envy and gratitude

MARCO CHIESA

Envy is a universal and ancient concept, which has been present within the culture of all known civilizations in the history of time. The deeply rooted impulse to begrudge others' better fortune and the wish to spoil for others what we do not have is also well documented in religion and in literature. The juxtaposition between Hell and Heaven, devils and angels depicts the constant battle between the destructive and the creative forces present in human nature. This theme is powerfully portrayed in Milton's *Paradise Lost*, in which Satan's envy of God' s attributes and of Heaven lead him to wage war on God (Milton, 1975). Eventually Satan and other allied angels are expelled from Heaven and they build Hell as the place where the destructive attacks against God's creations can be planned and carried out. In Shakespeare's *Othello* (Shakespeare, 1969) the main protagonist, blinded by his own furious jealousy, ends up murdering the person he loves. In the same play – although Shakespeare does use envy and jealousy interchangeably – he describes envy as 'the green-eyed monster which doth mock the meat it feeds on'. He also makes reference on the inborn component of envy 'they are not ever jealous for the cause, but jealous for they are jealous; 'tis a monster begot upon itself, born on itself '.

In *The Divine Comedy* Dante Alighieri (1954) places the envious souls in the second circle of the Purgatory. Their punishment is to wear coarse hair-cloths and to have their eyes stitched with wire. The eye, the sight has a special importance as the sense organ that stimulates envy, and through which envy operates, as the expression 'to cast an evil eye upon somebody' testifies. It is interesting to note that by not placing the envious souls in Hell Dante believes that they can be purged and obtain purification.

In addressing female sexual development Freud describes the wish for girls to possess the male genitals as a way to compensate for feeling castrated (female castration complex). The realization of the difference with male genitalia leaves the girl in a state of grief and resentment for having been deprived of that organ. The girl holds mother responsible for her lack of a penis and she turns to father in the hope that he will endow her with a penis in the shape of a baby (Freud, 1917). Freud believes that penis envy is very important for development and character formation, and that it may lead, unless resolved, to sexual inhibition, to neurosis or to an intensification of masculine traits in the girl character structure. Freud also holds that penis envy plays a crucial role in shaping the Oedipus Complex. However, Freud does not recognize other forms envy may take and does not extend the concept to other dimensions of psychic life. In addition an unfortunate inference from Freud's work is that envy seems specifically confined to the female gender.

Abraham gave an important contribution to the psychoanalytic conceptualization of envy. He ascribed some states of chronic neurotic resistance to the analytic process to the presence of elements of envy towards the analyst (Abraham, 1919). Central to his thinking was the narcissistic injury inflicted by the awareness that the analyst may possess knowledge and skills that the patient needs to improve his condition. The patient responds to such awareness with hostility and with the desire to spite and devalue the analyst's possessions. He considers the female castration complex in the light of an injury occurring during the narcissistic phase of the girl's development, when she harbours avaricious-hostile feelings of wanting to deprive the other person of what she herself does not have (such as male genitalia) (Abraham, 1920). In a subsequent paper Abraham (1921) traces the origin of envy in the oral-and-anal-sadistic stage of development.

Envy and gratitude

Klein is the author who, more than anyone else, has addressed and broadened the significance and manifold functions envy has in shaping psychic development and in structuring the personality. Envy has a central role in Kleinian thinking, which enhances our understanding of the internal and external manifestations of human destructiveness. Although Klein referred to envy in her early work, she gave her most extensive contribution on the role played by envy later in life (Klein, 1957). This is the result of the coherent progression of her work based on the centrality of the conflict between death and life drives, and within this the death drive is seen as the cornerstone, which underpins the paranoid-schizoid position and her general theory of anxiety. Klein's conceptualization of envy provoked strong disagreement and criticisms among many analysts (Spillius, 1993), who did not accept the idea that envy could be constitutionally rooted in the human being (Joffe, 1969). In addition it created a misconception in other schools of thought that Kleinian analysts were too preoccupied with destructiveness to the detriment of other aspects in the clinical situation.

Klein extended Freud's notion of penis envy to encompass other manifestations of infantile psychic life such as the child's phantasized attacks on mother's possessions like the paternal penis or the babies contained in her abdomen (Klein, 1928; Klein, 1932). In *Envy and Gratitude* (1957) she describes in detail the central features of envy, conceptualized as the direct expression of the destructive impulses specifically directed against the source of life. The original object of the destructive attacks is the mother's breast, the very source of the child's nourishment and gratification. In intrauterine life the unborn baby has uninterrupted and unlimited supply of sustenance via the maternal placenta. After birth the baby, who has in his mind a phantasy of an inexhaustible breast, has to cope with the inevitable frustration that the breast may not be available exactly when it is needed to satisfy his hunger. Klein postulated that object relationships, however rudimentary they may be, are present from birth and that frustration and gratification are experienced in relation to an object (see Chapter 8). The baby's experience of the absent breast as a malevolent object inflicting pain and hurt on to him triggers feelings of hostility towards the depriving and frustrating object.

Although early experiences of deprivation and other traumatic environmental experiences are important factors in enhancing and stimulating envy, Klein makes it clear that the envious attacks are fundamentally directed towards the good and gratifying primary object, and not against the bad and frustrating breast. The good object is resented and hated because it is endowed with life-giving qualities, which the baby depends on for his survival. The baby gradually realizes that the source of good experiences of feeding and comforting is an external object. Under the influence of envy the baby wishes first to possess the good qualities of the object and then, when he realizes that this is unobtainable, to attack and spoil the good experience and the object itself. Envy also seeks to place badness into the object in the form of bad excrements and bad parts of the self; this process is accompanied by the phantasy of freeing oneself of one's destructive impulses. The spoiling of the good experience results in great difficulties in taking and keeping inside one's mind (introjecting) good and benign objects. The violently attacked objects are turned into damaged and vindictive objects, which are then internalized as such. Internal bad and persecutory experiences cannot therefore be balanced and counteracted by the presence and operation of good internal objects. Attacks on the good experience lead to further complications. After the good experience is turned bad the baby feels deprived, which leads to further attacks against the object now blamed for the deprivation and for keeping the goodness to itself. A vicious circle is thus established whereby envy destroys the goodness of the object, leading to deprivation and persecution, which in turn increase the hatred towards an object now experienced as mean and sadistic.

It seems important to be aware that not all attacks on the breast and on the primary object are motivated by envy. Early and severe physical and emotional traumas arouse states of helpless rage, which may lead to the experience of loss of the good experience. The effect on development and the adult clinical manifestations of long-lasting frustration deprivation and lack of maternal empathy with the infant's agonizing mental state has been particularly studied by Rosenfeld (1978, 1987a). He emphasizes the importance of differentiating between destructive narcissistic patients in whom constitutional factors such as envy are prominent, from traumatized borderline patients in whom destructive attacks against the object originate from severe early environmental failures. It seems important to bear in mind that the relationship between, and mutual influence of, envy and early repeated traumas are not yet fully understood, as in the not uncommon cases in which they are both prominent factors in clinical presentation.

Envy is considered to be strongly associated with negative therapeutic reactions, that is a worsening of the patient's mental state following a period of improvement or relief after sessions. Although other interrelated factors such as unconscious sense of guilt (Freud, S. 1923; Riviere, 1936), a need for punishment, the operation of the death instinct (Freud, S. 1937) are relevant to the understanding of negative therapeutic reactions, here I will focus on the role played by envy. When the patient feels reached by the analyst's interpretations and experiences relief, he may unconsciously feel resentful of the analyst's capacity to understand him. The patient may react in such a way to destroy the work done jointly with the analyst, in fact often denying that any good work has ever taken place. It is not unusual that interpretations of the negative therapeutic reaction are followed by amnesia of what occurred in previous sessions. The often-silent attacks towards the analyst are an expression of the subject's unconscious hatred that the analyst has something useful to offer, which the patient needs. By reaching the patient and offering understanding that benefits him, the analyst implicitly challenges the patient's devaluation of him and his omnipotent phantasies of superiority over the analyst. In addition helpful interventions threaten to expose the patient's dependency on the analyst and his need for a good object. As Rosenfeld (1987b) points out, the envious attacks are not only directed against the good experience with the analyst but also against the part of the patient who needs and receives help. Therefore envy undermines parts of the ego as well as external and internal objects. The persistence of excessive oral envy leads the patient to incorporate the 'good' analyst omnipotently and to identify with him. This takeover allows the patient to believe that he is the source of the good experience, and that he, not the analyst, has done the good work.

Since envy interferes with the early process of splitting between the good and the bad object, it becomes a powerful source of confusional states. As Klein clearly described, excessive envy is an obstacle to the introjection of the good object, which becomes spoilt under the influence of envious attacks. Consequently the normal split between the good and the bad internal object (see Chapter 3) cannot occur sufficiently, which paves the way for later disturbances in differentiation between, and recognition of, good and bad experiences. Love and hate, good and bad cannot be kept apart. Rosenfeld applied these discoveries to the understanding and treatment of acute confusional states in psychosis, the severity and duration of which he attributed to the strength of inborn envy. He further described that psychotic patients build up elaborated schizoid defences against the experience of confusion. These defences drive them away from any meaningful contact that may evoke a strong emotional reaction leading to a confusional state (Rosenfeld, 1950, 1964). Klein also suggests that confusional states may be used defensively to obscure awareness of the envious attack and of the damage inflicted on the object.

Since excessive envy systematically attacks and damages the good object, the envious person feels unable to have good experiences, and gratification and enjoyment are minimal. The experience of deprivation strengthens the destructive attacks on the object, which result in a vicious circle with envy, deprivation and introjection of mean and ungiving objects reinforcing one another. The resulting failure to introject good and benign objects seriously weakens one's capacity for love. The relative lack of gratification undermines the feelings of love for an external object capable of providing pleasurable, satisfying and fulfilling experiences.

The repeated gratifying experiences at the breast outweigh destructive, hostile and anxiety-laden elements and reinforce a sense of deep-seated love and gratitude for the object. The presence and experience of the 'good breast', which satisfy the child's instinctual and emotional needs, are the building block for a solid relation with the good object and underlie the appreciation for the goodness in others and in oneself. It is through the integration and identification with a solidly introjected good object that the individual develops a spontaneous sense of generosity and trust, rooted in the wish to share with others the good experiences he himself received (see Chapter 4).

Gratitude is an indispensable pre-condition for developing the capacity to make reparation, and for sublimatory activities to take place. When envy and external frustration are not excessive the child is able to develop a sense of enjoyment, a capacity to experience pleasure. The child develops awareness that there is a caring and loving external object, capable of unselfish and dedicated care. The introjection of such an experience linked to a giving object enables the child to bear the imperfections and shortcomings of the caregiver, and to develop a sense of tolerance and forgiveness. Under these circumstances the child's reparative capacities are considerably strength- ened and can easily be mobilized when the object has been the target of the child's attacks. When hostile and persecutory anxieties temporarily predom- inate, the child is able to draw from the immediate external response of the object and from the internalized experience of the good breast to weather the storm and to regain the link with the good object. This relieving experi- ence of a 'new dawn' reinforces appreciation and love for the good object. Excessive envy interferes with the introjection of the gratifying experience and consequently thwarts the development of a trusting and grateful relationship with the object. The not uncommon experience in analytic practice of patients who find it difficult to thrive from their analysts' strength and help, while holding on to grievances for their inevitable failures and mistakes may be rooted in the operation of envy. Petot (1991) states, 'It is the conceptualization of the interest in the object as gratitude, necessary to the perfection of gratification, which is the most decisive development. It is inseparable from the formation of a theory of the introjection of the good breast, which seems to be the organizing principle of Melanie Klein's later ideas' (p. 200).

Relationship between envy, jealousy and greed

In everyday language and sometimes in literature envy is often associated with, and mistaken for, jealousy. In fact jealousy is a less primitive emotion connected with a relationship between three people; therefore its onset dates back to the Oedipal situation. Jealousy is concerned with a fear of losing one's loved object to a third party. The wish is not to deprive or spoil for someone else the good experience and the good object, as it is the case in envy, but to retain it for himself. In the early Oedipal configuration the dawning awareness of a third figure, the father, creates anxieties in the child that he may lose his privileged position with the primary object, the mother, and be excluded by the parental couple. Jealousy is more motivated by love than by hatred, even though in pathological forms jealousy can become very consuming and lead to controlling behaviour, dangerous and destructive actions. At times envy can operate in a disguised form in triangular liaisons, where the primary aim is to create pain and deprivation in the third person, rather than obtain the good experience/object for oneself. For example, the compulsive Don Giovanni, who seduces a married woman, but quickly loses interest and drops her when he succeeds, creates destruction and devasta- tion for both husband and wife. Since envy, jealousy and greed are closely bound with each other, it is often difficult to draw a clear differentiation between their ubiquitous clinical manifestations.

Greed refers to the strong wish to possess what is intensely desired and needed. In the infantile situation the hungry baby latches on to the breast, yearning for milk, suckling greedily with no pauses; in these circumstances breast-feeding can be a painful and trying experience for the mother. Greed though is an emotion that goes far beyond the satisfaction of one's needs. The drive is to take rapaciously everything the object has, with no concern for the state in which the object is left. Greed is at the source of primitive phantasies to empty the breast of all its goodness and leave it dry. Because in greed something good in the object is recognized and because the main aim is not to spoil but to want it for oneself, it is thought that libidinal and destructive components operate in a balance.

Defences against envy

Envy is a pervasive emotion whose destructive effects hamper development. It is therefore an experience that is highly difficult to recognize in oneself. Powerful and complex defences are built to ward off awareness of it.

Primitive idealization keeps the primary object so high up on a pedestal that it cannot be reached. The ideal object is so idolized that it is kept in a different planet, so out of range that it does not elicit envy, as if it does not belong to this world.

The presence of devaluation of the self may be employed to cover envy directed against the object. Often a type of masochistic self-debasement is held on to tenaciously. The circular and relentless nature of self-devaluation is such that either the other person stops existing or is kept immobilized as an impotent spectator. In this way any envy of the object is obliterated.

At the opposite end inflation of one's capacities and values creates a self-belief that everyone else is inferior and that they wish to rob him of the attributes he believes he is endowed with. Therefore envy is projected into the object and then it is experienced as directed against the subject (see Chapter 9). Elaborate strategies may be employed to actually stir envy in others. Consequently the subject feels surrounded by envious objects and the fear of being attacked can lead to delusional developments associated with paranoid ideation. The object may be subject to intense attacks and criticisms aimed at devaluing it. The lack of recognition of the value of the object may be defensive against experiencing envy, as a devalued object does not elicit envy.

As Klein states, the defences against envy are manifold and often operate in synergistic cooperation. A patient, Ms A, tended to idealize me and she showed overt appreciation of the progress achieved during analysis, while any feelings of hostility and grievance were directed against external objects. Her praise of me did not seem to square with her repeated lateness for sessions, her increasing silences and overall withdrawal from contact. She wished to end treatment at short notice due to external circumstances and because she felt that she had 'gone as far as she could go in the analysis'. She continued to deny any negative feelings towards me and the analysis, until a dream, in which I was portrayed as a failing and incompetent schoolteacher, revealed her contempt and devaluation of me, and her lateness, silences and wish to stop could be understood as attacks on the analysis.

Defences against awareness of envy can have a handicapping effect on the personality development and substantially limit the extent of progress in analysis. Such defences are never successful and split-off envy always operates in a disguised, but nonetheless destructive form against creativity and development. The combination and synergic operation of these multiple defences may establish a system that operates as a pathological organization of the personality (Steiner, 1993).

Clinical illustration

Mrs H was thirty-four when she came into analysis, following two serious attempts to take her life, for which she had been hospitalized. She was an introverted and chronically depressed woman, who spoke very little in short and condensed sentences that were at times barely audible. She idealized death as a solution to the difficulties and disappointments of life, and as a means of inflicting to herself a final retribution for her own failings and shortcomings. Her wish to be dead permeated almost every session, which, alongside her overall retarded and withdrawn posture and her long and heavy silences, created a deep atmosphere of deadness and stagnation. Mrs H tried to wrap me, and recruit me, into her suicidal world. During the first weeks of analysis she dreamt of me prescribing her cyanide tablets, for which she was very grateful as she felt that this gesture was a proof that I understood her predicaments.

I will describe material from three consecutive sessions following a Christmas break, in her third year of analysis after Mrs H had made substantial improvements in her external and, to a degree, internal life. Mrs H broke the silence unusually quickly to mention that her husband George seemed to be more worried than herself that she made it to the session on time. She explained that she was woken up by her 18-month-old baby daughter Rosy at 4.30 a.m. and had stayed on the sofa bed in her room. At 6.45 George went into the room to make sure Mrs H was awake. After a pause she reported a dream she had during the holidays.

> I was in central London with Rosy and George, and we were heading for a station or a shopping centre. George though decided to go somewhere else on his own, and Rosy followed him. I assumed that George would notice that Rosy had gone after him and consequently that he would look after her. When George returned

alone, I realized that Rosy must have got lost. I became very anxious and I started
to look for Rosy with no success: I felt that I had lost her for good. I felt very
distressed and anxious at the thought of having lost Rosy, but the other people
around me in the dream seemed to be unconcerned and calm.

She thought that the dream might be connected to her discovery during the
holidays that she was pregnant: she feared a repeat of the miscarriage that
occurred nine months earlier. I interpreted that the dream scenario was a
reflection of her experience of the holiday break: a part of her felt very
alarmed and distressed while the Mrs H present in the sessions before the
break had felt unconcerned and detached. Her reply was to say that she was
so preoccupied with the preparations for Xmas that she had no time to think
about the break. She had hosted a number of relatives over Xmas and was so
worried that everything fell into the right place. She mentioned that she had
given herself away to her relatives by not drinking alcohol during the festiv-
ities, and she had to let them know that she was pregnant. She did not want
to break the news so early on, so as not to tempt faith. I pointed out that she
feared that she might give something away to me regarding how she might
have felt not to have sessions during the Christmas break. She then 'loses' the
part of her (Rosy) in the dream that felt abandoned and vulnerable, which
allows her to take on a detached position.

The session continued with Mrs H bringing lively material about the situation in her family as she was concerned that her older sister Jane did not get
on with her father, and how caught in the middle she felt. After a pause she
said that she was feeling guilty now for having spoken of internal family
affairs. She felt as though she had betrayed her family and did not want me to
think that she was being disloyal. She locked herself into an uneasy silence in
the remaining five minutes of the session.

The following day Mrs H was nearly ten minutes late. After a while I
commented on her silence, to which she replied, 'I have said too much
yesterday.' After more silence she said, 'This will have to come to an end soon
... maybe at the end of the spring or in the summer.'

After a pause she snapped, 'It is very difficult when you do not give me a
response to what I have just said.' I described to her the withdrawn and
coldly hostile state of mind she had come to the session with. After a pause I
said that after she had been open and had brought the news of her
pregnancy, something in her had turned against it by the time the previous
session was drawing to an end.

Mrs H responded with a mocking remark: 'Yes, this is the usual pattern ...
you should be used to it by now.' The session continued with silences inter-
spersed with almost inaudible fragments of sentences. In the third session of
the week Mrs H started in a similar withdrawn and silent state. She recalled a
dream:

> I was witnessing an exchange between my sister Jane and my father from which I inferred that things were much more on a friendly footing between them. I felt relieved and I conveyed my impression to Jane, who replied that in fact nothing had changed and that she and father were still on a warpath. I felt deflated and disappointed.

Mrs H said the dream showed that once again she had got it wrong, that her impressions of what was going on between her sister and her father must be incorrect. She should not make wrong inferences otherwise she will end up disappointed. I reminded Mrs H that in the Wednesday session she had been open, had told me about the pregnancy and had felt that we were getting on well. Then a Jane part of her takes over and convinces her that nothing of the kind really happened on Wednesday, that she should be, and always will be, her usual cold and withdrawn self. I also showed her how she had turned away from the experience of a good contact with me to a more hostile and distancing part of herself.

Mrs H recalled a second dream:

> I am at the bottom of a staircase; I look up and see that my nephew Nick has opened the stair-gate. Rosy, who is alongside Nick, makes a move to come down the stairs. I fear the worst but I manage to intervene just on time and I take Rosy in my arms.

Mrs H said that in reality something similar happened over Christmas when her sister's family were guests of Mrs H. She was very busy and had not realized that Nick, who was upstairs with Rosy, had opened the stair-gate and was encouraging her to go downstairs. Luckily she walked past the stairs at that precise moment and prevented what could have been a serious accident. Later in the session she spoke about a documentary that she had seen the previous evening centred on a woman who had suffered a nervous breakdown. After discharge from hospital she was allocated an aide who helped her emotionally and practically to resume normal life. This woman did not appreciate the help received though. In fact she unearthed and destroyed the plants that the aide helped her to plant in her garden.

Of course the material presented may be looked at from different angles. What I would like to emphasize here is the shift that occurred between the first and subsequent sessions. In the first session Mrs H was unusually open and communicative. She seemed in touch with feelings of anxiety and loss as present in the dream of losing Rosy, she allowed a dialogue between us to take place and seemed to be receptive to my interventions.

In that session Mrs H broke the news of the pregnancy she had longed for following the miscarriage nine months previously, after which she had been very anxious about her ability to conceive again. Mrs H had spoken with unaccustomary freedom about her internal family affairs, bringing details of the difficult relationship between her sister and her father. As the session drew to a close, though, a change occurred within her, expressed as 'her guilt' for betraying her family for revealing too much to me. She then withdrew into silence. Here Mrs H turns away from the Rosy part of herself, representing the infantile aspect, which wants to be in contact with her father (myself in the transference). Mrs H attacks the connection established with me in the first part of the session and her happiness and relief for having conceived. She becomes the Jane of her dream, cold, distant, hostile and destructive of our work, which defiantly says that nothing has really changed. Clearly Mrs H's destructive attack on the good experience is increased by the weekend separation in which I become the abandoning George who does not keep in mind the Rosy/Mrs H who does not want the week to end. Although the interpretation of the attacks on the analysis helps her to retrieve the Rosy part of her, as shown in the dream in which she saves Rosy from falling down the stairs, Mrs H identifies with the ill patient of the documentary who does not appreciate the help received and destroys the work of the aide.

Discussion

The relationship between envy and the primary instincts has been the object of discussion over the years but, in my opinion, conceptual clarity has not yet been fully achieved. Klein points out that envy is the outward manifestation of the death instinct, but in a different passage she notes that envy is rooted in need and admiration. Segal mentions that envy 'arises from primitive love and admiration', and that it 'has less strong libidinal component than greed and is suffused with the death instinct' (Segal, 1973). It seems that envy is seen as an ambivalent emotion in which libidinal or destructive forces may predominate (Segal, 1993). There is still some lack of clarity over whether envy should be considered a direct manifestation of the death instinct, subsequently mitigated, outweighed by, and suffused with, the life forces; or whether it should be conceptualized as stemming from primary love and admiration, but immediately infiltrated and taken over by primary destructiveness; or again whether it results from a specific merger between manifestations of the death and life instinct.

If we take a look beyond the couch at the history of humanity, at the manifestations of these primitive emotions in the social dimension, this may give us important additional understanding. There seems to be general agreement that greed has greater libidinal components than envy does, as the primary aim is to obtain the goodness felt to be possessed by the object, and not to find pleasure in spoiling whatever good the object may have. The inference is that greed carries less destructive potential than envy. Yet if we look beyond the individual to the social manifestations of these primitive emotions, we are inclined to the view that greed has exerted as devastating blows to humanity and to the environment in which we live as envy has.

Historically genocide has been motivated by the insatiable hunger for possession of land, natural resources and riches 'owned' by a different race. The systematic massacre of entire civilizations (for example the Incas, the Aztec and the Mayas in Latin America, and the Red Indians in North America) rested upon greedy appropriation of territory for the victors' consumption as well as upon the desire to destroy out of envy of a different culture. More recently the insatiable thirst for oil of western civilization has been one of the major motivating forces for the Gulf War and the need to create an emasculated protectorate in the Middle East.

Envy entails a two-person relationship mostly based on an internal wish that something bad happens to the other person, consistent with its Latin origin ('to cast an evil eye upon'), to draw enjoyment from somebody else's misadventure or failure, to feel a sense of begrudging resentment for someone else's success. The human and environmental exploitation and destruction is based as much on greedy, selfishly inexhaustible hunger for resources for oneself at the expenses of others, as on a wish to deprive and spoil it for others. Nations wage wars for supremacy, for the control of territory and of natural resources as well as on the primitive persecutory anxiety of being overpowered and dominated by the enemy, and by the predominance of psychotic processes at group level (Segal, 1997a).

Although Chaucer describes envy as the worse sin of all, 'for all the other sins are sins against one virtue, whereas envy is against all virtue and against all goodness', Dante places envious sinners in Purgatory and sinners of greed in the Inferno. Therefore he regards greed as a worse sin than envy. In reality envy, jealousy and greed do not operate independently in a pure form, but a considerable degree of overlap of the three emotions is invariably present in clinical manifestations of human behaviour.

The relative weight and influence on personality development attributed to envy derived from inborn drives and to early environmental experiences is still a lively topic of debate. Klein emphasized the inborn nature of envy, the genetic loading of which varies for each individual. Nevertheless she stressed the impact of the trauma of birth, of early frustrations at the breast and of inadequate mothering as important factors which increase the intensity of envy. Equally repeated favourable external experiences may outweigh and counterbalance the operation of inborn envy. Clearly the particular individual circumstances and the idiosyncratic balance between internal innate and external environmental factors, and the complex interaction between them, will determine the outcome in each individual case. Klein regarded the outcome of personality development in this area as dependent on the balance between three factors: (1) constitutional intensity of envy, (2) constitutional strength/weakness of the ego, and (3) external favourable/ unfavourable environmental circumstances, such as the quality of caregiving.

However, in clinical practice it is often impossible to have a clear and unequivocal picture of what the early environment had been like for the patient. We have to rely on the, at times contradictory, conscious recollections brought by the patient, on the unconscious communication derived from internal primitive object relations, and on our countertransferential responses and our intuitive understanding of the material to reconstruct what the patient's early environmental experiences might have been. This poses a technical challenge in our interpretative work of patients' negative manifestations in the clinical encounter. Specifically we need to understand the extent to which these negative reactions may represent manifestations of envious attacks against the analytic work, or be ascribable to other factors, such as the re-enactment of early emotionally traumatic relationships with primary objects. In the latter case the infant may be subjected to maternal projections and to frequent misunderstandings of his emotional state. These repeated environmental failures might lead to the accumulation of unexpressed narcissistic rage in the subject's unconscious, which may never find expression. In these cases over-interpretation of envy creates in the patient a feeling of being misunderstood and criticized by the analyst, and lead to an impasse (Rosenfeld, 1987b).

The following material is drawn from a case I supervised. The patient, Ms B, entered three-times-a-week therapy after a once-weekly spell in the National Health Service, where she had been originally referred on account of depression and poor self-image. Her mother, who had had a very difficult relationship with her own mother, found it hard to cope with the demands made by the three children and with an unfaithful husband. She became depressed, attempted to take her life through overdose and was twice admitted to hospital. Ms B and the other two children were sent to stay with neighbours for a few weeks. Ms B experienced these early separations as traumatic rejections and as evidence that mother could not cope with her and did not love her. Ms B reported instances which indicated that a degree of physical and emotional traumas had been inflicted to Ms B by both parents. As it became clear soon after the start of therapy, Ms B showed considerable contempt for anyone who was nice to her and she repeatedly attacked any good experience she received from the therapist or from external objects. She was in a relationship with a gentle and giving boyfriend, but she was often cruel to him and pined for a previous boyfriend who had 'always behaved like a bastard'. The initial emerging picture consisted of a blend of early environmental traumatization, complex identifications with a cruel primary object and intermittent envious reactions.

The session I am going to present occurred in the week preceding the Christmas break. Ms B had cancelled the previous session because of ill health. She started the session with a familiar string of complaints about how terrible her life was and how she did not deserve anything better anyway. She felt lonely and isolated. She mentioned that her boyfriend Mike spoke to her about his plans for a two-week holiday next summer. Ms B was nasty to him in return, and made it clear to Mike that there was no point in planning so far ahead since they may not be together come the summer. An attempt by the therapist to link the material with the forthcoming two-week break was dismissed as irrelevant by the patient. The therapist reported to me that she felt increasingly unsympathetic, bored and distant from the patient.

She took up the destructiveness enacted by Ms B in her relationship with Mike, wondering whether something similar was happening in the session, with reference to Ms B's missed session. After a silence the patient reported that she had felt unwell, went to see her GP, but her urine sample was found to be clear. She later developed a high temperature, returned to the surgery, a urinary tract infection was diagnosed and she was prescribed antibiotics. Ms B felt angry with the GP who took a careless view of the patient and did not listen to her. At this point the therapist interpreted the patient's anger with her for taking a break. Ms B had telephoned her mother the evening before with a view to find out what had happened during her childhood, to try and clarify her confused memories and experiences. Her mother said that she always loved Ms B but that she was such an awful child, and put forward a series of unclear reasons to justify her own failings. She added that Ms B's emotional problems should be put down to genetic inheritance, as her own mother and brother had also suffered from depression. Ms B felt more confused than at the beginning of the conversation, and indeed her state of mind was clearly conveyed to the therapist, who felt herself uncertain as to what to do in the session. Ms B was clearly affected by the forthcoming inter-ruption of treatment perceived as a cruelty inflicted upon her as evidenced by her complaints of isolation, by the reference to the two-week summer holiday, by her having fallen ill two days earlier, and by her cruel treatment of Mike. However the therapist's first attempt to reach her was rejected, and she became annoyed with the patient, feeling that nothing worthwhile could be achieved in the session, given the patient's state of mind. From then on the therapist's few interventions addressed Ms B's destructiveness in a rather non-specific way.

With hindsight we could reach a different understanding of what had occurred in the session. Ms B tried to convey how she had wanted to find out from her mother what went wrong in her childhood and what was wrong with her health from her GP, but how both of them failed her. Ms B tried to convey her confusion and unbearable state of mind to the therapist who in identification with the patient's mother, was experienced as blaming the daughter/patient for her own failings. The therapist might have interpreted that Ms B was experiencing her like her GP, not really listening and not taking on board her experience of frustration and confusion, and that she felt she was with a person she was unable to get through to; in other words that Ms B was with an object experienced as uncaring and impervious. In these circumstances it is helpful not to emphasize the patient's destructiveness, which the patient experiences as blaming and critical, just like her own mother had been during the telephone conversation.

This case shows how early and sustained environmental difficulties intertwined with innate envy form a complex clinical picture of negative manifestations in the therapeutic encounter. A balanced approach to interpretative work, a close monitoring of counter-transferential reactions and a fine-tuning to the details of verbal and non-verbal material in the transference are required in order to understand and reach the patient.

CHAPTER 8

What are internal objects?

CATALINA BRONSTEIN

Introduction

The terms 'internal object' and 'internalized objects' are currently widely used in psychoanalysis. Even though the concept of 'internal objects' was present in Freud's writings, it was Melanie Klein who developed this concept and made it central to her theory of psychic functioning. Klein refers to 'internal objects' and to the relationship with and between 'internalized objects' throughout her work.

The concept of 'internal objects' covers a multiplicity of psychic phenomena and therefore lends itself to confusion. When we think of the word 'object' as that to which the subject relates, we are mostly describing someone or something that has an emotional meaning for the individual. This can be seen to entail in Segal's words: 'almost the totality of our emotional experience' (Segal, 1999, p. 96). In order to disentangle the different ways in which this concept is used it is important to look first at its development in Freud's work.

Historical

The concept of 'object' in Freud is intimately linked to the concept of 'drive'. The object is mainly seen by Freud as the thing 'in regard to which or through which the instinct is able to achieve its aim' (Freud, 1915a, p. 122). Freud distinguishes between the object of the sexual drive and its aim: 'Let us call the person from whom sexual gratification proceeds the sexual object and the act towards which the instinct tends the sexual aim' (Freud, 1905b, pp. 135-6). The object becomes assigned to the drive 'only in consequence of being peculiarly fitted to make satisfaction possible' (Freud, 1915a, p. 122). It is what is the most variable about the drive and it is not originally connected with it. Freud suggests that it seems probable that the sexual drive is, in the first instance, independent of its object (Freud, 1905b). This seems to imply that, for him, the choice of object is determined more by the history of each individual subject than by constitutional factors (Laplanche and Pontalis, 1973).

In his paper 'On narcissism: an introduction' (1914) Freud introduces an important idea: that of the ego becoming the object of libidinal desires. He describes how certain individuals may chose their love-objects according to a model based on themselves, that is, 'seeking themselves as a love-object' (Freud, 1914, p. 88). He is describing the ego here both as a functioning apparatus and as an object. In 'Mourning and melancholia' (1917), Freud extends the concepts discussed in his paper on narcissism. He introduces a different view of the relationship to the object as well as placing the emphasis here more on the object than on the drive. It was mainly these developments that particularly influenced Klein's thinking.

In 1911 Abraham published a paper where he described some similarities between the normal process of mourning and severe depression (Abraham, 1911). Freud extended and developed these ideas in his paper 'Mourning and melancholia' (1917) where he described the importance of *identification* in states of melancholia. While in ordinary mourning the world seems to become poor and empty, in states of melancholia it is the ego that suffers that fate. The melancholic state is one where there is a reaction to the loss of a loved object, but where the object has not died, but has been lost as an object of love. The melancholic is full of self-reproaches which Freud deduces are reproaches against the loved object that had been taken into the ego which is now identified with the object: 'Thus the shadow of the object fell upon the ego' (Freud, 1917, p. 249).

One of the questions that Freud seems to be trying to answer is how this mechanism of identification is carried out. Freud relates the mechanism of identification to the oral instinctual impulse of *incorporation* (following Abraham), and to the mental counterpart of this oral impulse, or *introjection* (following Ferenczi) (Sandler, 1987). He sees introjection as forming the basis of identification, though he does not always keep the two terms apart. It seems important to note that he is suggesting that the process of identification is the first form of attachment to another person:

> ... what is called an 'identification' – that is to say, the assimilation of one ego to another one, [i.e. to an object] as a result of which the first ego behaves like the second in certain respects, imitates it and in a sense takes it up into itself. Identification has been not unsuitably compared with the oral, cannibalistic incorporation of another person. It is a very important form of attachment to someone else, probably the very first, and not the same thing as the choice of an object. (Freud, 1933b, p. 63)

Ferenczi had already introduced the concept of *introjection* in 1909, contrasting it with the mechanism of projection used by paranoid patients:

> Whereas the paranoiac expels from his ego the impulses that have become unpleasant, the neurotic helps himself by taking into the ego as large as possible a part of the outer world, making it the object of unconscious phantasies ... One might give to this process, in contrast to projection the name of Introjection. (Ferenczi, 1909, p. 47)

He later describes it as 'an extension to the external world of the original autoerotic interests, by including its objects in the ego' (Ferenczi, 1912, p. 316).

Abraham describes how in melancholia the loss of a loved person is succeeded by an act of introjection which has the character of a physical incorporation by way of the mouth (cannibalistic) (Abraham, 1924), implying that there is a regression to the oral phase. This conceptualization exercised an important influence on Melanie Klein's ideas.

The use of the concept of 'object' does not just comprise the real external object, or its perception, but in as much as it produces an identification of the ego with the object, the object is felt to form part of the ego. It could be therefore said that the process of internalization has an organizing effect on the mind, a structuring role (Merea, 1980) and that the processes of introjection and identification are integral to the development of the ego. In 'The ego and the id' Freud states:

> When it happens that a person has to give up a sexual object, there quite often ensues an alteration of his ego which can only be described as a setting up of the object inside the ego, as it occurs in melancholia ... It may be that this identification is the sole condition under which the id can give up its objects. At any rate the process, especially in the early phases of development, is a very frequent one, and it makes it possible to suppose that the character of the ego is a precipitate of abandoned object-cathexis and that it contains the history of those object-choices. (Freud, 1923, pp. 29-30)

Freud proposes that, in melancholia, once the object has been introjected by the ego it is now judged by a special agency as if it were the forsaken object. The melancholic self-reproaches would then be reproaches to the part of his ego identified with the hated object. Therefore, the conflict between the ego and the lost loved person is transformed into a conflict within the ego. The ego becomes split into two pieces; one, an agency Freud called 'conscience', a critical agency within the ego and which he describes as 'among the major institutions of the ego' (Freud, 1917 (1915b), p. 247), raging against the part of the ego identified with the lost object, that is: 'the one which has been altered by introjection and which contains the lost object' (Freud, 1921, p. 109).

The critical agency is named as the 'superego' in 'The ego and the id', where Freud writes that those early identifications (which he links to the dissolution of the Oedipus Complex) may be taken to form a precipitate in the ego: the superego (Freud, 1923, p. 34).

Internal objects, the life and death drives and the integration of the ego

The proposition that identification with objects affects the structure of the ego was taken up by Klein. However, Klein's concept of internalized objects is more extensive than the idea of object-cathexis. When we think of the concept of 'internal objects' as part of a Kleinian metapsychology, we have to think of it in the context of its interaction with other main hypotheses, such as: the existence of life and death drives, a theory of early mental functioning which formulates the existence of an ego capable of perceiving anxiety, the development by the ego of primitive defence mechanisms, the hypothesis of unconscious phantasy and the theory of paranoid-schizoid and depressive positions (Bianchedi, 1984). One can say that Kleinian theory is both a drive and an object relations theory.

In Klein's view the mechanisms of *projection* and *introjection* are basic to the constitution of the ego and there is an intrinsic connection between them (see Chapters 3, 9 and 11). This means that if the infant attributes his own loving and hateful feelings to the breast, the experience he takes back in will be coloured by these projections:

> By projection, by turning outward libido and aggression and imbuing the object with them, the infant's first object-relation comes about. This is the process which, in my opinion, underlies the cathexis of objects. Owing to the process of introjection, this first object is simultaneously taken into the self. (Klein, 1952a, p. 58)

Introjection is considered by Klein as the mental activity by which the child, in his phantasy, takes into himself everything he perceives in the outside world. Given that the child's main satisfaction comes initially via the mouth, she deduces that the child will use the mouth in phantasy to incorporate the world. Even though the mouth is the main channel, the other sensory channels also 'take in' the world outside him. The emotional state that enables the baby to incorporate a good experience, such as pleasure at the breast, in both its satisfying qualities of satiation of hunger and of sexual pleasure is stressed by Klein:

> The first gratification that the child derives from the external world is the satisfaction experienced in being fed. Analysis has shown that only one part of this satisfaction results from the alleviation of hunger and that another part, no less

important, results from the pleasure which the baby experiences when his mouth is stimulated by sucking at his mother's breast. This gratification is an essential part of the child's sexuality, and is indeed its initial expression ... To begin with, the breast of the mother is the object of his constant desire and therefore is the first thing to be introjected. (Klein, 1936, p. 291)

The ego in Kleinian theory is present and active from the beginning of life and establishes relations with objects from the first contacts with the external world (see Chapter 11). Klein's idea of the first object, the 'mother's breast', should not be taken in a strict literal way as it represents the mother as felt by the baby in his first contact with her, whether the baby is being breastfed or not. Klein proposes that the infant concretely internalizes the breast and the milk it gives. This process is experienced by the infant in a primitive way, not yet mediated by language. She further clarifies this, noting that the breast is not just a mere physical object. The breast is imbued by the infant's unconscious phantasies and desires with loving qualities that go beyond the nourishment it provides (Klein, 1957):

We find in the analysis of our patients that the breast in its good aspect is the proto-type of maternal goodness, inexhaustible patience and generosity, as well as creativeness. It is these phantasies and instinctual needs that so enrich the primal object that it remains the foundation for hope, trust, and belief in goodness. (Klein, 1957, p. 180)

According to Klein, the workings of the life and death drives include their attachment to objects from the beginning of the infant's life. She sees the process of introjection working mostly in the service of the life drive, enabling the ego to take in something life-giving and thus binding the death instinct working within (Klein, 1958). However, this is not the only function that this mechanism has: the ego introjects both 'good' and 'bad' objects. The object (mother's breast is the prototype) becomes bad because the baby projects its own aggression on to it. The re-introjection of the breast containing the projected hostility leads to the unconscious phantasy of a 'bad' internal breast within the ego. This creates a 'phantastically distorted picture', in the ego of the infant, of the real object upon which the maternal object is based (Klein, 1935).

The first objects experienced by the baby are 'part' objects (such as the breast) and are split between 'good' and 'bad'. This corresponds to Klein's description of the paranoid-schizoid position. The 'bad' breast is felt to be bad not only because it frustrates the baby (for example when it does not satisfy his hunger), but also, as has been mentioned above, because the baby projects his own aggression into it (Klein, 1935, p. 263). (Note that 'good' and 'bad' should be always thought of as relative terms and put in inverted commas, to show that their qualities have been attributed subjectively by the infant (Laplanche, 1981).) The 'good' breast becomes the prototype of what is felt throughout life to be beneficent, helpful and loved, while the 'bad' breast stands for what is persecuting and hated. Klein's description of the early 'good' and 'bad' internal objects is intended to capture the infant's very early experience of the world which cannot be put into words. This very primitive experience is felt concretely in bodily form. Money-Kyrle describes this as a stage where no distinction is made between the representation and the object represented, in which the infant sustains a concrete belief in a physically present object (Money-Kyrle, 1968, p. 422). For example, a hungry baby is thought to experience the object as a 'bad' one, located in his tummy. These 'part objects' are felt to be 'whole' by the baby and are experienced in a concrete way, following bodily sensations, either pleasurable or painful. This world of unconscious omnipotent phantasies of a concrete quality persists in the individual and can resurface, for example, in dreams (Hinshelwood, 1989, pp. 73–4).

We need to specify here that there is a certain ambiguity in Klein's use of the concept of ego. She sometimes uses it to describe the whole personality, more akin to what we would describe as 'self', while at other times, the term ego retains the original meaning in the 'structural' sense as the agency of the personality in charge of a number of particular functions (Spillius, unpublished paper).

The role of anxiety, and its intimate connection with the state of internal objects (and thus the ego), occupies a central position in Kleinian thinking. Klein put forward the hypothesis that the primary cause of anxiety is the fear of annihilation of life, which arises from the death instinct within. Given that in the child the ego has not attained full development, he is very much more under the influence of his unconscious. Klein believed that the greater or lesser cohesiveness of the ego at the beginning of life was linked to its capacity to tolerate anxiety, which she thought was a constitutional factor (Klein, 1946, p. 4). The struggle between the life and death drives, which emanates from the id, involves the ego, and the danger of being destroyed by the death instinct gives rise to the first defence mechanisms (see Chapter 3). Even though Klein recognizes the influence of frustration in generating hostility in the baby, she finds the principal source of hostility to be the death instinct:

> We may assume that the struggle between life and death instincts already operates during birth and accentuates the persecutory anxiety aroused by this painful experience. It would seem that this experience has the effect of making the external world, including the first external object, the mother's breast, appear hostile. To this contributes the fact that the ego turns the destructive impulses against the primary object. The young infant feels that frustration by the breast,

which in fact implies danger to life, is the retaliation for his destructive impulses towards it and that the frustrating breast is persecuting him. In addition he projects his destructive impulses on to the breast, that is to say, deflects the death instinct outwards and in these ways the attacked breast becomes the external representative of the death instinct. The bad breast is also introjected, and this intensifies, as we may assume, the internal danger situation, i.e. the fear of the activity of the death instinct within. (Klein, 1948, p. 31)

From this we can see that among the ego's first activities are the defences against anxiety (experienced initially as persecutory anxiety) via the use of the processes of splitting, projection and introjection (Klein, 1952a, p. 57; see also Chapter 3). It seems clear though that introjection of the good object is not only a defence mechanism against anxiety but also an intrinsic part of the libidinal relationship to the breast.

Splitting of the object (and of the ego) into good and bad is one of the first defence mechanisms which the ego employs to deal with anxiety, while projection is the primal process of deflecting the death instinct outwards. In 1946 Klein introduced the concept of projective identification as a defence mechanism by which part of the ego is attributed to an object and thus disowned (Klein, 1946, p. 8). Post-Kleinian analysts have deepened the understanding of this defence mechanism (see Chapter 9). The term 'project-ive identification' is now widely used and often replaces that of 'projection' as it brings together the defence mechanism with the unconscious phantasy of the consequences to both self and object.

In Klein's view, the primal 'good' object forms 'the core of the ego' (Klein, 1957, p. 180), it 'acts as a focal point in the ego' (Klein, 1946, p. 6). This first 'good' internalized object counteracts the process of splitting and dispersal, making for cohesiveness and integration. The more the mother and her breast are cathected, and this in part depends on the baby's inherent capacity to love, the more securely will the internalized 'good' breast become in the infant's mind (Klein, 1955a). Klein sees the ego as developing largely round the 'good' maternal object, while the identification with the good aspects of the mother becomes the basis for further helpful identifications (Klein, 1959b, p. 251). This has been underlined by Rosenfeld, who proposed that phantasies and feelings about the state of the internal object vitally influence the structure of the ego (Rosenfeld, 1983).

One of the primal functions of the ego is its drive towards integration. Similarly as with splitting, the concept of integration includes that of the object as well as of the ego. This involves a movement from part-objects towards whole objects in the depressive position (see Chapter 4). We can assume that the movement from part-objects to whole objects, that is, towards an integrated ego, is not an even one, and is influenced by the strength of the life drive as well as by internalization of good objects. This implies in some measure the 'acceptance by the ego of the working of the death instinct':

> The more the ego can integrate its destructive impulses and synthesize the different aspects of its objects, the richer it becomes; for the split-off parts of the self and of impulses which are rejected because they arouse anxiety and give pain also contain valuable aspects of the personality and of the phantasy life which is impoverished by splitting them off. (Klein, 1958, p. 245)

The strength of the ego was seen by Klein to reflect the state of fusion between the two drives (which she felt was partly constitutionally determined), that is, between love and hate. If in the fusion, the life drive predominates, there is a greater capacity to love and the ego is more able to bear the anxiety that arises from the death instinct and to counteract it (Klein, 1958, p. 239).

The vicissitudes experienced by both object and ego give rise to the different types of identification characteristic of the two positions: paranoid-schizoid and depressive and to the fluctuations between them (see Chapters 3, 4 and 5). We can see a type of 'narcissistic' identification in the paranoid-schizoid position, in which the individual feels that bad internal objects are separate from himself but acting as tyrants over him, while at other times he becomes identified with the internal tyrants or persecuting objects. This describes the case of internal objects virtually assimilating the ego. However, it can also be felt by the self and seen by the analyst as the ego taking over the object. In such an experience the boundaries between the subject and the object are blurred and the subject does not distinguish between himself (or part of himself) and the object. The subject might then feel confused and trapped in a hostile internal world and might compulsively try to rid him/herself of the persecuting experience. An example of this could be seen in a disturbed 18-year-old adolescent girl, whom I will call Emma. She was tormented by persecuting nightmares in which she was trapped in a room full of mirrors which reflected her image at different ages, some of which could not be discriminated from her mother's image. Emma had attempted suicide several times and had once attacked her mother with a knife. She sought some sense of relief through cutting herself, which she pursued until she drew blood and experienced pain. She explained her self-harming behaviour as the only possible 'solution'; it was the only way she could achieve a sense of being 'herself'. But this 'solution' was one brought in by hatred of herself (in her identification with her mother), and instead of appeasing her sense of 'badness' it increased her persecutory guilt and her sense of despair.

Another type of identification can be seen in the depressive position where the independence of the object is recognized and identification is thus different in quality. In it the separateness of object and self and their relative wholeness are recognized. The subject becomes 'like' the object rather than 'being' the object. (I. Sodre, 'Who's Who', unpublished paper; E. Spillius, unpublished paper). For example, an adolescent girl may see herself as a potential future mother and as having good, loving, maternal capabilities in identification with these same aspects in her own mother, without either needing to deprive her real mother of these qualities or becoming confused with her. This type of identification takes into account the existence of an 'I' or 'me' as distinct from the 'internalized objects', as well as a 'good' maternal internal object free to have a sexual life of her own.

Internal objects and unconscious phantasy

In one of her descriptions of the dynamics of internal objects in the ego Klein states:

> In my experience, there is, furthermore, a deep anxiety as to the dangers which await the object inside the ego. It cannot be safely maintained there, as the inside is felt to be a dangerous and poisonous place in which the loved object would perish. Here we see one of the situations which I described above, as being funda- mental for the 'loss of the loved object'; the situation namely, when the ego becomes fully identified with its good internalized objects, and at the same time becomes aware of its own incapacity to protect and preserve them against the internalized persecuting objects and the id. ... We know that, at this stage, the ego makes a greater use of introjection of the good object as a mechanism of defence. (Klein, 1935, p. 265)

We can see here that Klein looks at the concept of 'internalized object' in two ways. First, she describes how the internal object forms part of the ego through introjection and how this is used as a defence mechanism. Secondly, she refers to an unconscious phantasy of the inside as a dangerous and poison- ous place where the good objects may perish.

It seems helpful, following Baranger, to elaborate on Klein's use of the idea of internal objects from these two different perspectives. In the first, internal objects play a role in the development of the ego and superego; that is, in the structuring of the agencies of the personality; this can be called a metapsychological viewpoint. In the second perspective, internal objects are looked at descriptively, which Baranger calls a phenomenological dimension (Baranger, 1980). The phenomenological aspect can be seen in the phantas- matic qualities that internal objects can acquire, such as having an intention and an independent life of their own, for example, in the phantasy of a poison- ous attacking breast or in the destructive power of the baby's urine. There is therefore a certain ambiguity in the concept of 'internal objects', which at the same time allows greater versatility.

According to Baranger (1980) the internal objects underlie a multiplicity of phenomena and affective states which are conditioned by them. Consciously, they appear to us through images, memories, dreams, of an infinite variety. This was also stressed by Sandler and Sandler (1998), who saw internal objects as being evident only in the shape of their derivatives (dreams, daydreams, actions etc.). They can express themselves in several different forms, for example a persecuting object can come into view as part of night terrors, daydreams, as well as in phobias. Bion introduced an important new perspective to the theory of internal objects in stating that the part-object relationship in the paranoid-schizoid position is not with an anatomical part only (that is the breast), but with a function, 'not with anatomy but with physiology, not with the breast but with feeding, poisoning, loving, hating' (Bion, 1959). We can therefore see how, in phantasy, the internalized object is experienced as having intentionality.

This shows us that, for Klein, internal objects cannot be thought of separately from either the mechanisms that create them or the underlying unconscious phantasies (see Chapter 2). Unconscious phantasy and internal objects can be defined as being in a dialectical reciprocal relationship (Baranger, 1980). They come together as part of the same psychic experience. It seems to me that it is theoretically helpful to maintain a distinction between unconscious phantasy and internal objects. However, given the experiential basis of Kleinian theory, internalized objects are often seen to *be* unconscious phantasies.

When we think in terms of unconscious phantasies, it becomes more difficult to use a structural model, since unconscious phantasies permeate the whole of the psychic apparatus. It might be clearer to think more in terms of more or less primitive unconscious phantasies, taking into account that they are all derivatives from the life and death drives. The degree of 'unconsciousness' also varies. Klein assumes that unconscious phantasies are experienced by the baby in a very concrete way; therefore she describes unconscious phantasies in bodily terms as she thought this was the way the baby feels:

> The baby, having incorporated his parents, feels them to be live people inside his body in the concrete way in which deep unconscious phantasies are experienced - they are, in his mind, 'internal' or 'inner' objects. (Klein, 1940, p. 345)

Internalized objects can adopt, in phantasy, any form, as well as relating to each other. In an undated manuscript in the Melanie Klein papers where she tries to describe what she means by internal objects and the contrast with the classical concept of superego, she writes:

My reason for preferring this term to the classic definition, that of 'an object installed in the ego' is that the term 'inner object' is more specific since it exactly expresses what the child's unconscious, and for that matter the adult's in deep layers, feels about it. In these layers it is not felt to be part of the mind in the sense, as we have learnt to understand it, of the super-ego being the parents' voices inside one's mind. This is the concept we find in the higher strata of the unconscious. In the deeper layers, however, it is felt to be a physical being, or rather a multitude of beings, which with all their activities, friendly and hostile, lodge inside one's body, particularly inside the abdomen, a conception to which physiological processes and sensations of all kinds, in the past and in the present, have contributed. (D16, Melanie Klein Trust papers, Wellcome Library) (quoted in Hinshelwood, 1997)

From this we can gather that the same term 'inner object' has been used to convey different experiences in the infant, which range from the very early, concrete, pre-verbal bodily experiences to more sophisticated ones. It is used to describe an unconscious phantasy of containing either a friendly or hostile being as well as its status as an integral part of the development of the ego and superego.

The process of splitting of the breast and ego confronts us with one of the paradoxes in relation to this formulation, as we always move on two separate but interrelated planes. On the one hand, Klein sees the ego as a centre of functions (capable of perceiving anxiety, and splitting the object), on the other, as being structured round the object, in identification with it. Internalized objects can acquire, in Klein's view, a status of not belonging to any distinct part of the psychic apparatus. This is where their phenomenological status becomes clearer. She states for example, that in the process of mourning, after working through the feelings of hatred, guilt and triumph caused by the death of a loved person, the individual can achieve a state of greater freedom in the inner world which enables him to pine for the lost loved object, leading to a situation in which 'internalized objects, being less controlled by the ego, are also allowed more freedom' (Klein, 1940, p. 359). It is as if the ego then gives greater freedom to the internalized objects, enabling them to go through a variety of feelings, allowing them to be separate, even to confront each other.

The child's anxiety about his ego and his internal objects is one of the incentives to check and understand the external world as a way to calibrate his internal world: 'The visible mother thus provides continuous proofs of what the "internal" mother is like, whether she is loving or angry, helpful or revengeful' (Klein, 1940, p. 346). This shows that for Klein, perceptions of external reality are used to prove or to disprove anxieties concerning internal reality. The characteristics of internal objects as distinct from the external ones can be seen in the sometimes rigid and prohibitive quality of the child's superego. This concept had already been introduced by Freud and expanded by Klein. Klein does recognize the importance that the external object has on the infant's emotional development, such as the mother's handling of her baby, her capacity to understand him and the impact of both gratifying and frustrating experiences on the infant. Even though she did not neglect the impact that the external world and the relationship with parents had on the infant, her main aim was to focus on the subject's psychic reality. Bion added an important contribution through his exploration of the role that the mother's actual capacity to contain anxiety has on the psychic development of the child (see Chapter 12).

'Internal objects' are not only present through the baby's external encounter with the mother. According to Klein, the infant has an unconscious awareness of the existence of the mother (Klein, 1959b, p. 248). The internal object appears for Klein at a point of interconnection to a multiplicity of unconscious phantasies, which are part of what she sees as the child's inheritance. This idea was further developed by Bion in his postulate of the baby being born with a pre-conception or state of expectation of the breast (Bion, 1963). When the pre-conception of the breast is brought together with a realization of an actual external breast, the outcome, according to Bion, is the conception of the breast. This mating of the a priori knowledge of the breast with the experience of satisfaction produces a 'conception' of the breast. But this is still not a 'thought'. In order for thought to develop the infant has to experience the mating of the pre-conception of the breast with the experience of frustration and absence of the breast, described by Bion as a 'no-breast' (Bion, 1959, 1962b, p. 111; see also Chapter 12). What happens next, he says, depends on the infant's capacity to bear frustration.

Internal objects and superego

The concept of the superego and its connection with that of 'internal objects' is a complex one. Klein was not a neat theoretician and her ideas about the superego reflect this. The superego appears in her writings at times as a function rather than as an agency, as in the 'structural' model; at other times she sees the superego as an 'internal object' (see Chapter 11).

During the analysis of Rita, who was two years and nine months old, Klein came across the little girl's intense feelings of guilt. Rita presented with a marked inhibition in her capacity to play, night terrors (*pavor nocturnes*), a dread of animals, inability to tolerate deprivations and an excessive fixation on her mother, contrasting with great ambivalence towards her. The outbreak of her neurosis coincided with the birth of her brother. Klein realized that there was a strong connection between the development of

Rita's neurosis and the Oedipus Complex, which she saw as experienced even at such an early age. Rita's hostility towards her mother expressed itself in her unconscious desire to take the baby away from her, even during pregnancy, causing the child to suffer from intense anxiety and guilt (Klein, 1926). Guilt was then linked to the development of the Oedipus Complex, which Klein then saw as starting at a far earlier age than originally thought by Freud (see Chapter 6). Her view of the timing of the emergence of the superego, as well as its source, diverged from Freud's view and it was one of the points of contention between Melanie Klein and Anna Freud.

Klein sees Rita's inhibition in play as originating from her sense of guilt:

> Analysis showed that she did not dare to play at being the mother because the baby-doll stood to her amongst other things for the little brother whom she had wanted to take away from her mother, even during the pregnancy. But here the prohibition of the childish wish no longer emanated from the real mother, but from an introjected mother, whose role she enacted for me in many ways and who exercised a harsher and more cruel influence upon her than her real mother had ever done. (Klein, 1926, p. 132)

Klein adds here that what she is describing corresponds to what is known as the superego in adults. She thinks that the effect of this infantile superego weighs more heavily than the adult one because of its effect upon a weaker, infantile ego. The other reason for the harshness of this early superego is its connection to the pre-genital phases of development (the oral and sadistic phases) as described by Abraham (1924).

Initially Klein suggested that the superego came into being when these phases were in the ascendant and that explained its sadistic activity (Klein, 1928). She was at this time putting forward the idea that the structure of the superego was:

> built up of identifications dating from very different periods and strata in the mental life. These identifications are surprisingly contradictory in nature, excessive goodness and excessive severity existing side by side. (Klein, 1928, p. 187)

According to Hinshelwood (1989, p. 100), this reference shows how for Klein there are multiple constituents of the superego which are varied and endowed with specific functions in phantasy, as that of a vengeful devouring object, a primitive controlling object etc. At this time she called these internalized paternal figures 'imagos' and proposed that psychoanalysis played a vital role in diminishing the anxiety aroused by the superego's severity, opening the way for development of more 'kindly imagos' (Klein, 1929, p. 209). We can see that modification of the harshness of the superego was an important clinical consideration for Klein. This idea gains strength later on when she develops her theory of the depressive position (see Chapter 4).

In 'The early development of conscience in the child' (1933) Klein states that the:

> person's conscience is a precipitate or representative of his early relations to his parents. He has in some sense internalized his parents – has taken them into himself. There they become a differentiated part of his ego – his super-ego – and an agency which advances against the rest of his ego certain requirements, reproaches and admonitions, and which stands in opposition to his instinctual impulses. (p. 248)

In the small child, the super-ego has the most bizarre and phantastic character. This internal representative of the parents is created out of imaginary pictures of them formed not only of their own nature but also by the child's projection of his own impulses into them. The child then takes this distorted perception of the parents into himself and it may not coincide with the picture presented by the real parents. For example, a child's phobic anxiety may be based upon his fear of his own superego and/or his fear of real external objects which are now viewed in a phantastic light under the influence of his superego.

In the above paper (Klein, 1933) she links the superego with the aggression linked to the death instinct. She asks herself why some children form such monstrous and phantastic images of their parents. In cases where the child's sadism is very intense the infant experiences the danger of being destroyed by the instinct of aggression and experiences overwhelming anxiety. Klein sees the early sadistic superego as an offshoot of very intensive destructive impulses. The child displaces the source of his anxiety outwards, by projecting it on to external objects who become dangerous, creating more fear and anxiety and setting up a vicious circle by which the child is impelled to attack the object, thus creating even more anxiety. She states:

> analysis can never do away with the sadistic nucleus of the super-ego which has been formed under the primacy of the pre-genital levels; but it can mitigate it by increasing the strength of the genital level, so that the now more powerful ego can deal with the super-ego. (Klein, 1933, p. 256)

We can see here that Klein was proposing the idea that a superego of a milder type was one governed by the genital level but that the internal conflict with sadistic aspects of the superego is never completely resolved.

Klein maintained that the formation of the superego 'begins at the same time as the child makes its earliest oral introjection of its objects' (Klein, 1933, p. 251). At first, Klein, following Freud, linked the formation of the superego to the Oedipus Complex. However, in as much as she wrote of an early Oedipus Complex, the superego was also seen as originating very early (see Chapter 6). When she later described the Oedipus Complex in connection to the depressive position, she maintained the relative independence of the superego from the Oedipus Complex and kept it as originating very early:

> the super-ego precedes by some months the beginning of the Oedipus Complex, a beginning which I date, together with that of the depressive position, in the second quarter of the first year. Thus the early introjection of the good and bad breast is the foundation of the super-ego and influences the development of the Oedipus Complex. (Klein, 1958, p. 240)

It seems to me that the disconnection of the origin of the superego from the Oedipus Complex gives rise to a less precise formulation in Klein than in Freud. In Klein's thinking the concept of superego is thought about sometimes as structure and sometimes as function. With the formulation of the depressive position in 1935 and the strengthening of the theoretical influence of internal objects, the superego becomes a concept describing mainly internal objects that have a harsh and critical character (Hinshelwood, 1989, p. 104).

> The ego, supported by the internalized good object and strengthened by the identification with it, projects a portion of the death instinct into that part of itself which it has split off – a part which thus comes to be in opposition to the rest of the ego and forms the basis of the super-ego. (Klein, 1958, p. 240)

However, Klein also adds that the superego is not just the receptacle for the deflected death drive. It also contains the deflected portions of the life drive that is fused with it.

> Along with these deflections, parts of the good and bad objects are split off from the ego to the super-ego. The super-ego thus acquires both protective and threatening qualities ... As the process of integration – present from the beginning in both the ego and the super-ego – goes on, the death instinct is bound, up to a point, by the super-ego. (Klein, 1958, p. 240)

Klein therefore stresses that superego formation involves fusion of the drives. This is clinically important as in melancholic states the de-fusion of the death drive may be regarded as making the superego carry the ego to its own destruction. The role played by destructive impulses in the development of an extremely harsh, cruel superego, whose omnipotence can be idealized, and its links to psychopathology, has been a matter of interest to a number of post-Kleinian analysts, such as Bion (1959), Rosenfeld (1952), Brenman (1985), Riesenberg-Malcolm (1999) and O'Shaughnessy (1999).

A brief example of the struggle between loving and aggressive feelings towards internal objects is that of Mr D, a young man in his thirties who spent the first years of his analysis blaming his parents, mainly his mother, for his own difficulties. His relentless reproaches towards his parents were easily converted into self-reproaches which he dealt with by victimizing himself, thus resulting in a vicious circle of blame and punishment. For quite a long time in his analysis he had no apparent awareness of how painful it was for me to witness his repeated attacks on himself and on my efforts to help him. When he started to become more able to feel concern and bear painful feelings, he produced the following dream: 'there was a little girl on a fence. She wanted me to pick her up. I picked her up but she was like an inanimate woman, like a doll and very fragile. I held her with great care, trying not to harm her.'

He brought associations in connection to a five-year-old girl with whom he played some sexual games when he was about 10 years old. At that time he had felt abandoned by his mother who was an alcoholic and needed frequent hospital admissions. He expressed concern that he might have harmed the little girl beyond repair. This was linked by him to an experience with his mother (who had died several years ago) when he had once tried to feed her and she could not possibly take in any food. Mr D showed pain, concern and guilt while recounting this dream. This was very different from previous dreams, which were mostly felt to be persecuting. One could say that the little girl might represent his mother in the dream, a vulnerable and fragile mother who stirred up powerful feelings of sexual excitement, as well as of hatred for her neglect and guilt for the death wishes he had towards her, and that this was now experienced in the transference (where the woman in the dream could be seen to represent his mother-me). But we could also see the dream as a representation of the way his ego is functioning at a particular point in the analysis. The little girl/mother could then represent an abused and consequently fragile aspect of himself, a part of him that is now feeling more able to recognize his need for help as well as his capacity to care for his objects and who is trying to repair the damage he feels he has done to them, in particular to his mother. This dream could be seen as a communication to me that I should be very careful in the way I handle his now more available loving feelings as they could easily get destroyed by him. I was made aware that he was still sitting on the fence (still relying on his 'de-fences').

Klein stresses the importance of integration, which she sees as integration of the destructive impulses with more benign impulses and as a synthesizing of the different aspects of its objects by the ego. Integration is achieved in the depressive position and is based on the preponderance of the life instinct and implies the acceptance by the ego of the working of the death instinct. This can be seen clinically in the move from a very persecuting and harsh super ego in the paranoid-schizoid position to the development in the depressive position of a capacity to repair the damage done in reality and in phantasy to his objects so that the individual feels able to experience more love and gratitude towards them. It leads to a 'world of people predominantly at peace with each other and with the ego, inner harmony, security and integration' (Klein, 1940, p. 345), with more trust in inner goodness, a better capacity to contain anxiety and to relate to external reality as well as a greater freedom in the internal world.

CHAPTER 9

Projective identification

DAVID BELL

Introduction

In 1946 Melanie Klein published a short paper entitled 'Notes on some schizoid mechanisms' in which she summarized an important part of her work to date. In this paper there are a number of important conceptual innovations which include: the articulation of those anxieties and defences that constitute the paranoid-schizoid position, the recognition that it is not only the object that is altered by splitting processes but the ego itself, the distinction between binary splitting (that is, for example, splitting that results in a separation between 'good' and 'bad' aspects of the self and object) and a more violent activity which results in fragmentation and annihilation of parts of the self.[1]

Although the concept of projective identification is not the principal focus of the paper, it is the starting point for a huge output of literature on the subject. Elucidation of this concept has been one of the main growth points of contemporary psychoanalysis. The term has come to cover a number of phenomena which are quite distinct and as Sandler (1983) has pointed out, such elasticity of psychoanalytic concepts is inevitable. However, much is to be gained from differentiating the different processes to which the term refers, and it will be the aim of this chapter to draw out these distinctions.

Historical

Freud used the term projection to refer to a number of related but distinct mental processes, but central to them all is the relocation of mental contents

---

[1] The concept of splitting of the ego was an important preoccupation among psychoanalysts at this time, a testimony to the importance of Freud's 'Splitting of the ego in the process of defence', published posthumously in 1940.

on to the representation of the outer world. Something that was internal is now viewed as existing in external space, much in the sense that an image is projected on to a screen.[2]

In classical psychiatry the mechanism of projection has long been known to be central to paranoia. Here the subject attributes to an object in the outside world feelings or wishes that he repudiates in himself. Thus, for example, the recognition by a patient of his own sexual impulses causes anxiety. To defend himself against this anxiety the impulses are disowned and projected onto a figure in the outside world. As a result, the patient experiences another as trying to force himself upon him sexually. So what starts off life as a conflict between the ego and an instinctual impulse resolves itself into a conflict between the ego and the outside world.

Example

An acutely paranoid patient tried to keep a distance between himself and all other patients on the ward. If any man touched him he would shout defiantly 'I am not queer.' A wish to maintain psychological distance from his own homosexual feelings has been concretized into a need to maintain geographical distance from the patients on the ward who are felt to contain the repudiated impulses.

Similar mechanisms underlie phobia formation where the phobic object is felt to contain threatening parts of the self. The recognition of the centrality of the mechanism of paranoia to various types of mental pathology is already clear in Freud's earliest writings (see for example Freud, 1895, 1896) where he discusses the adaptive consequences of the mechanism of projection. According to Freud, the ego is threatened basically by two categories of stimulation – that which arises from the outside and that from the inside. Stimulation from the outside can be dealt with through the taking of defensive action (e.g. flight), but there can be no flight from the threat of internal (instinctual) stimulation. However through the location of the impulse externally the subject derives the advantage that he can evade the impulse through his evasion of the object into which it has been projected.

In 1910, in the paper on Leonardo da Vinci[3] , Freud describes a projective process which is closer to our theme. Freud believed that central to Leonardo's psychic world was his need to maintain in his mind a particular relation with his mother, namely one in which he feels himself to be loved by her with the inten-

---

[2]Freud was loosely influenced also by the use of the term in neuroanatomy where one speaks of the 'projection' of sensory fibres onto the cortical surface.

[3]This paper makes considerable biographical claims many of which have been repudiated, though this is not relevant to the point I wish to make which is purely theoretical.

sity of devotion. Unable to give up his mother as the central object of his libidinal life and unable to maintain it in full consciousness because of the conflict that it instigates (for example the fear arising from rivalry with the father) the problem is resolved through the ego's ancient ways of dealing with the impossibility of renouncing an object of its desire – it retains the object through incorporating it, becoming it, in other words through identification.

> The boy represses his love for his mother: puts himself in her place, identifies himself with her, and takes his own person as a model in whose likeness he chooses the new objects of his love. In this way he becomes homosexual [...] (Freud, 1910a, p. 100)

This complex psychic re-arrangement I would argue pre-figures the processes which we today describe as projective identification. The subject (in this case Leonardo) has taken his mother inside himself, he has become identified with her. His own infantile self has been projected into the young men who have become the object of his erotic interest and through treating them with such devotion he is able to maintain, unconsciously, the central relationship between a devoted mother and her son. From the perspective of consciousness Leonardo loves boys whom he regards as distinct from himself. But from an objective point of view his erotic objects are aspects of himself and it is for this reason that Freud states in the same paragraph:

> He finds the objects of his love along the path of *narcissism*, as we say; for Narcissus, according to the Greek legend, was a youth who preferred his own reflection to everything else and who was changed into the lovely flower of that name. (Freud, *op. cit.*, p. 100)

I will return later to the relation between narcissism and projective identification.

Freud goes on to say that each time Leonardo turns towards a woman and then replaces her in his mind with a man he repeats the 'mechanism by which he acquired his homosexuality'.

Note that in describing these mental processes we use the word 'identification' in two ways that are quite distinct from each other and this has been the source of some confusion. When Leonardo projects his infantile self into the young men who become the object of his love, we say that Leonardo 'identifies' the boys with infantile aspects of himself, in other words he *attributes* to them characteristics which are really his own.[4] Here we use the word 'identify' in the sense of giving identity to, naming an object. When he,

---

[4]This immediately raises the question as to whether there is a distinction to be drawn conceptually between projection and projective identification and this is something that I will return to after discussing Klein's introduction of the term.

that is Leonardo, becomes his mother in relation to the young men he 'identifies' himself with her, in the sense of *acquiring* her characteristics.[5]

Klein's introduction of the term projective identification

In the 1946 paper Klein firstly summarizes her views on the early states of the ego. In the earliest phases of life the infantile mind organizes the world in such a way that those aspects of its world which are felt as 'good' (such as for example the mother who provides love, understanding and comfort) are radically separated from other aspects felt to be 'bad' (such as the mother who is absent who is experienced not as an absent object but as a persecuting, frustrating present object). In this way the infant's good objects, to whom he feels only loving feelings are protected from his hostile feelings now directed only towards the 'bad' object. This mental state, termed by Klein the 'paranoid-schizoid position', and defined as such for the first time in this paper, is dominated by the mechanism of splitting and projection, these mechanisms being brought into play to deal with very early anxiety situations (see Chapter 3). Klein expresses her debt to Fairbairn who independently used the term 'schizoid position' to describe exactly the same clinical phenomena that had arrested Klein.

Klein describes the infant's mind as internally menaced by frightening internal objects, this situation being dealt with by the mechanism of projection. As a result objects felt to be internal and threatening are re-located outside the self and so become the source of paranoid anxiety. Clearly before an object can be projected in this way, it must first be split off and thus paranoia and splitting processes are closely bound together. The state of mind dominated by these splitting and projective processes, Klein described as the 'paranoid-schizoid' position.[6]

Example

Mrs S creates within the analytic situation a rosy idealized atmosphere where she makes it clear that she regards her psychotherapist as far superior to the

---

[5]Britton (1998a, pp. 5-6) has drawn attention to this fundamental distinction between projective identification as attribution or acquisition. This will be discussed later in this chapter.

[6]It is important to note, however, that Klein differentiates herself from Fairbairn on two issues. Firstly Fairbairn believed that there was no internalization of a good object but only of bad objects, whereas for Klein the growth of the ego is centred upon the capacity to introject a good object that can support the ego in its development, such internalizations taking place from the beginning of life. Secondly, Fairbairn wished to abandon instinct theory for a purely object-relational point of view, whereas for Klein the interplay between the life and death instincts remained essential to her developmental model.

psychiatrist who she sees in the out-patient department of a psychiatric hospital. In one session she recounts how as a child, in order to escape from a very persecuting situation at home, she went out to the hills and holed up in a cave. There she 'painted over all the cracks in the walls of the cave with magic paint, to stop the monsters getting in'. Subsequently the therapist made an error as regards the age of one of her children. The atmosphere of the session suddenly changed and she accused the therapist of never having listened to her, of being useless and only interested in his own theories etc.

One might say that, in a way that reflected her childhood concerns, she had used the magic paint of idealization to turn the therapeutic situation into a protected retreat, all hostile feelings being directed elsewhere, towards the 'incompetent psychiatrists'. But as is the case with all idealization, the slightest crack, the error, caused a total collapse and the monsters, namely her own feelings of hatred and frustration, now had free access and overwhelmed any positive feelings

Klein also points out in this paper that it is not possible to split an object (say, into good and bad aspects) without their being at the same time a split in the ego. If one thinks about it, this must be so. For example in the state of being madly in love, the lover splits his object so that it has only good qualities, all its bad qualities being denied. But in relation to that object he has also split himself for he has only idealizing attitudes towards his loved object, these feelings being kept widely separated from any more hostile feelings. In 'Notes on some schizoid mechanisms', Klein brings out vividly the constant interplay between introjection and projection, the two fundamental dialectical movements of the mind. These movements take place in two locations, namely between the ego and its objects (i.e. still internal to the subject) and between the ego and the outside world. Impulses and objects projected externally are subsequently re-introjected and then re-projected, this being a constant movement throughout life. If the subject directs all his hating, biting and vengeful feelings towards an object he may suddenly feel persecuted by a vengeful hateful object that he has introjected and which is then felt to attack him internally, resulting in further projection. This understanding of the constant interplay between internal and external is central not only to Klein's model of the mind but also forms the basis of the clinical technique that she developed.[7]

---

[7]Klein saw the processes she was describing vividly illustrated in Ravel's opera The Magic Word (Klein, 1929). The child in the opera, after arguing with his mother about not wanting to do his homework, attacks various objects (these include smashing a teapot, trying to stab a squirrel and a furious attack upon a grandfather clock which involves removing the pendulum). The objects that have been attacked swell up and come to life and persecute him, but when he shows concern for a squirrel that has been bitten and binds the little creature's paw the world is restored to order.

It is important to differentiate between these 'micro' movements between internal and external and the more durable internalizations that are not so easily altered, that form part of what we call character. For Freud these more massive identifications did not take place until relatively late, that is with the internalization of the parental figures that form the superego, heir to the Oedipus Complex. For Klein and probably for most contemporary analysts these identifications long precede this relatively late developmental stage.

Now, returning to Klein's paper. There is something curious about the introduction of the term. From the historical vantage point that we now occupy one might reasonably expect the term projective identification to be announced in the paper as a new and fundamental discovery about mental life. But this is not the case. The term projective identification is introduced almost in passing for in many senses although the term itself is new the phenomena to which it refers have already been well described by Klein many years before.

Petot (1991) points out that what was new in the 1946 paper was not the concept of projective identification itself, but more in 'the possibilities it raises of relating introjection and projection as they appear in clinically observable manifestations, and as *they apply in turn to the same objects*' (Petot, 1991, pp. 164–5, italics in original).

Having summarized her views on introjective and projective processes, Klein turns more specifically to the infant's projection of bad aspects of himself into the primary object, normally the mother. Klein closely follows Freud's conception of the 'ego as first and foremost a bodily ego' (Freud, 1923) and so aspects of the self are always linked, psychologically, to parts of the body. Hated parts of the self, for example, are regarded as being identified with bodily excrement (though, of course, this is not an exclusive relation as elsewhere Klein makes it clear that the faeces can stand for many other phenomena, e.g. prized possessions, gifts to an object).

In the later 1952 version of the paper published in *Developments in Psycho-Analysis* the term 'projective identification' is introduced earlier in the paper and there is now a real sense of discovery. She says:

> Together with these harmful excrements, expelled in hatred, split-off parts of the ego are projected on to the mother, or as I would rather call it *into* the mother. These excrements and bad parts of the self are meant not only to injure but also to control and to take possession of the object. In so far as the mother comes to contain the bad parts of the self, she is not felt to be a separate individual but is felt to be *the* bad self. Much of the hatred against parts of the self is now directed towards the mother. This leads to a particular form of identification which establishes the prototype of an aggressive object-relation. I suggest for these processes the term 'projective identification'. (Klein (1946) in 1952, p. 300, italics in original)

It is important to emphasize that all the mental processes described refer to phantasies and thus the consequences described relate only to the subject. The effects on any actual external object, a preoccupation of later workers in this area, was not part of Klein's thinking at this stage.

Klein makes the point that it is, inevitably, difficult to describe these processes given that they occur at a time before the infant can think in words. It is also important to distinguish the point of view of the subject in whom these processes are occurring from our understanding of them, that is to distinguish the subjective from the objective point of view. When Klein says that the mother into whom these aspects of the self have been projected is now not a separate individual, that is she is now felt to be 'the bad self', this is, so to speak, from our more objective perspective. From the subject's point of view the 'bad' that has been projected is repudiated and it therefore appears to him as an object quite separate from himself, he *dis-identifies* himself from it.

It is clear from the above that here Klein is regarding projective identification as an aggressive action primarily with motives of control. However in the very next paragraph she points out that it is not only bad parts of the self that are projected but also good parts of the self and here it is perhaps hard to see this as essentially an aggressive mechanism.

Klein also, however, makes it clear that the mechanisms of splitting and projective identification provide vital protection for the internal good object and are therefore essential to development. It is only when these mechanisms are excessive and continue to dominate the functioning of the personality at later stages of development that the outcome is pathological. However Bion was later to point out that the type of projective identification that characterizes very disturbed mental states is not only excessive but also qualitatively different.

Klein draws out the effects on the subject's mental state that are consequent upon the use of these primitive mental mechanisms, by studying the fate of the projected objects in the external world (from the subject's point of view) and the consequences of projective identification for the inner world. She shows how these processes become the basis of some fundamental infantile anxiety situations.

First the projection of bad, hostile objects has the consequence that the subject feels menaced by these objects, now felt to be located in external space. As mentioned above, in Klein's first description of these processes she attributes two motives to projective identification which one might term specific and general. The specific motive for example may be to rid the self of a particular bad internal object or feeling[8], whereas the general motive appears in the way that the whole process effects a control of the object.

In the projective processes Klein describes it is not only the object that is projected but also the motive for projection. The subject who seeks to project bad aspects of himself into an object and through so doing to control the object subsequently feels menaced by hostile objects that are felt to be seeking to invade and control him. This mechanism frequently underlies claustrophobic anxieties.

Example

Ms C lies on the couch in every session in a state of terror and unable to move. In one session, after allowing the analyst to have more contact with her in a way that felt more benign she was able to tell her analyst that, as she walked behind him on her way from the waiting room to the consulting room, she felt irresistibly drawn to staring at his anal area in a way she clearly thought of as very invasive and threatening. It became clear that when she lay on the couch these invasive aspects of herself were now felt to be located in the analyst and she experienced him as boring into her with his eyes. She felt utterly controlled and unable to move.

On the other hand the projection of good aspects of the self results in the external object being idealized. The subject then feels himself to be entirely dependent on, indeed cannot live without the idealized object which is felt to contain all that is good. Klein, (drawing on the work of Paula Heimann, see Heimann, 1942), points out that this state of utter subservience to the idealized object comes quite close to a feeling of being persecuted by it.

Control appears to enter into the process of projective identification at another point. In phantasy, and as I will later describe, often in external

---

[8]We tend to talk rather loosely about projection of internal objects and projection of feeling states. Probably these are closely related, in that projecting an internal object felt to be bad creates a hostile relation between the self and the object of projection. Freud, as discussed above, described the projection of sexual impulses (that is, 'I feel sexual desire towards him' becomes 'he feels sexual desire towards me') whereas most Kleinians would also regard this situation as being brought about through the projection of internal objects. However there is a further complication, as Klein also describes the process of projection itself as being dominated by a feeling state (for example the infant may be regarded as projecting aspects of itself *in hatred* which, clearly, is not the same thing as projecting hatred). Rosenfeld defines projective identification in the following way: 'Projective Identification relates first of all to a splitting process of the early ego, where either good or bad parts of the self are split off from the ego and are as a further step projected in love or in hatred into external objects' (Rosenfeld, 1971b, p. 117).

reality, the object has to be controlled in order for the projective processes to be maintained.

Projection of parts of the self and of internal objects are, of course, phantasies, as parts of the mind cannot in reality be moved through space (see Chapter 2). Yet these phantasies have *real* effects on the state of the ego. If all aggressive feelings are projected into external objects this results in a real impoverishment of the ego. Projection of good aspects of the self similarly weakens the ego as in extreme states of romantic love where the lover feels himself to be but nothing before his beloved who constitutes all that is perfect in the world. The projection of lively good aspects of the self into other objects, leaving the self depleted, is also vividly described by Anna Freud (1937) in a process she calls 'altruistic surrender'. She describes a female patient who located the lively, enthusiastic and sexual parts of herself in others who she dutifully served, while she remained lifeless and impoverished.

States in which there is such wholesale projection of aspects of the self are termed schizoid states and are characterized by feelings of emptiness and unreality. Such patients often say they feel empty, unreal, as if something has gone missing. Klein's view would be that this is a perfectly accurate description of their state consequent on such massive projection.

A note on mechanism and phantasy

An important aspect of the above account which it would be easy to overlook, is that Klein is describing at one and the same time a psychological mechanism of defence and a particular type of unconscious phantasy. Namely there is a defensive process of projection and an unconscious phantasy that aspects of the self can be forced into other objects, to enter and affect those objects from within, altering them and controlling them. Implicit in this account is a conception of the mind as representing its own various functions through the means of unconscious phantasy. This was made most explicit in Susan Isaacs' seminal paper 'The nature and function of phantasy' (Isaacs, 1943). She points out that mechanisms, say the mechanism of introjection, are what we see, so to speak, 'from the outside', whereas unconscious phantasy describes what is experienced from the inside. For example, in the case of introjection there is a phantasy of taking aspects of the object into the self through a sort of psychic swallowing whereas, in the case of projective identification, the unconscious phantasy of forcefully ejecting aspects of the self follows the bodily model of vomiting or defecating.[9]

---

[9]The philosopher Richard Wollheim uses these concepts to discuss the way the mind represents to itself its own activities (see Wollheim, 1969).

Projection and projective identification

Some authors distinguish between projection and projective identification but from the account offered here this distinction does not hold. Projection is the mental mechanism whereas projective identification offers an account of the mechanism which includes the unconscious phantasy which is part of it. Spillius puts it thus:

> [British Kleinian analysts'] usual view, though rarely explicitly stated, is that it is not clinically useful to make a distinction between projection and projective identification. What Klein's concept of projective identification has done has been to add depth and meaningfulness to Freud's concept of projection by emphasizing that one cannot have a phantasy of projecting impulses without projecting part of the self, which involves splitting, and, further that impulses and parts of the self do not vanish when projected; they are felt to go into an object. Unconsciously, if not consciously, the individual retains some sort of contact with projected aspects of himself. (Spillius, 1988a, p. 82)

Some features of the state of mind consequent on the massive use of projective identification

Projective identification as described here cannot be thought of as an isolated mental mechanism but only in the context of those mental structures that constitute the paranoid-schizoid position.[10] The same mechanisms underlie clinical states which at first glance might seem so different. I have mentioned above that individuals who live in such a schizoid world often experience feelings of emptiness and unreality. Sometimes such people maintain themselves isolated from others who are unconsciously experienced as containing dreaded aspects of themselves. Alternatively as a result of projective identification the external object is felt to contain valued aspects of the self and this can result in compulsive clinging to the object, separation from it being felt as a catastrophic loss of part of the self. This is most obviously the case where the patient has projected 'good aspects' into others, but is not restricted to those cases.

Examples

1. A patient approaching a break described terrifying states of anxiety accompanied by fantasies of execution. This terror resulted from the

---

[10]Though we tend to think of projective identification only in the context of the paranoid-schizoid position some authors (for example Spillius, 1994) have pointed out that this mechanism is also the basis for empathy and where this is the case the projective identification described is more benign and part of a depressive world.

patient's having projected a large part of her own ego functions into the analyst and separation was therefore experienced as a violent disconnection from vital aspects of her own mind.

2. Another patient who habitually projected envious and greedy aspects of himself into others organized his life in such a way that he had constant access to others who were felt to embody these qualities, partly so that he could maintain his projective system but also at some level he recognized these aspects as truly belonging to himself.

In line with this it is a common finding in analysis that the reclaiming of even very distressing aspects of the self, despite the pain this inevitably brings, is accompanied by a worthwhile sense of integration.

As discussed above projective identification often results in terrors of being invaded and taken over or of being imprisoned. These processes are well illustrated in certain nightmare scenarios in popular films. For example in the film *Alien* the invading monster has the terrifying capacity to deposit embryonic parts of itself into the bodies of his prey. These embryos grow inside their host, take him over and destroy him.

A further feature common to the schizoid world is a pervasive sense of something being strange or altered in the world. This is frequently accompanied by an experience of the boundaries between the self and the outside world being felt to be very insubstantial. Such a world is felt to be full of looming presences and is accompanied by the sensation that in some mysterious way others know something about one, have special access to one's inner thoughts. This is the conscious counterpart to projective identification and in this sense it contains a certain truth. If I project aspects of myself into another person then, in this sense, that person is felt to have access to those aspects of my psychology that are now pictured as residing within him. Patients occupying a schizoid world often complain of feeling that they are not living their own life but instead feel as if they are playing a part in a play that someone else is directing. This again is the counterpart to the controlling aspect of projective identification; the person now feels he is being controlled by the objects of his projections.

Projective identification and psychosis

It will be apparent from the above that the processes being described have a close affinity with the phenomena described in patients who suffer from psychoses. Feelings of being invaded, taken over, of losing parts of oneself, of seeing the world as divided between enemies and saviours are part of the lived experience of these patients and are felt to be concrete events. Such a patient may experience the analyst's interpretation as robbing him of his thoughts or of trying to force aspects of the analyst's mind into the patient. The patient may feel that he has taken on the identity of a powerful other (e.g. Christ or God) and thus finds himself to be surrounded by envious others who seek to rob him of his powers.

The theory elaborated in 'Notes on some schizoid mechanisms', taken with the work that led up to it, in fact laid the foundation for a detailed understanding of both manic depressive psychosis and schizophrenia. As Klein put it:

> These various disturbances in the interplay between projection and introjection which imply excessive splitting of the ego, have a detrimental effect on the relation to the inner and outer world and seem to be at the root of some forms of schizophrenia. (Klein, 1946, p. 11)

In the appendix to 'Notes on some schizoid mechanisms' Klein gives a commentary on Freud's analysis of the Schreber Case (Freud, 1911b), where he gave his fullest account of a paranoid psychosis. Freud understood not only that Schreber's delusional world was based on the projection outwards of impulses and ideas of his own but that his descriptions were expressions of the state of his own ego. Thus, the idea that the world was coming to an end represented an accurate description of the state of his internal world, only projected externally. Klein develops this theme. Schreber's division of the world into good and bad is, as she put it, a 'projection of Schreber's feeling that his own ego is split, events which are entirely consistent with her theory. Though Klein herself did not analyse a psychotic patient[11] her analysands Segal, Rosenfeld and Bion all made this an essential part of their work and though these contributions differ widely, the elaboration of the concept of projective identification, and the working out of its implications for technique formed a central part of this work.

Development of the concept of projective identification in the work of Klein

The 1946 paper deals almost exclusively with the projection of parts of the self into objects but in the following years the same term is used to refer to something which is quite distinct, namely the projection of the self into an object. Through this process the self appropriates qualities of the object for itself. This wholesale identification of the self with the object is typical of psychotic states where the subject feels that he has become for example

---

[11]the child patient 'Dick' (see Klein, 1930) was probably autistic and so would these days be considered psychotic; however Klein did not analyse a schizophrenic or severe manic depressive case.

someone famous (such as Jesus), but in more subtle forms is part of common experience. Klein gives her fullest account of this form of projective identification in her paper 'On identification' (Klein, 1955a) where she uses a story by the author Julian Green to illustrate her theory. The story entitled 'If I were you' describes how the central character, Fabian, embittered with his own life and very envious of others, makes a pact with the Devil, whereby through uttering a magic formula in the ears of another he can exchange places with that person, take over his body and his life. He goes through a succession of such transformations and Klein follows meticulously his motives for the selection of each victim. A powerful motive underlying this violent taking over of another is, according to the story, envy. For example Fabian's first choice is to take over the body of his employer who he imagines as fabulously wealthy and '[who] can enjoy life to the full ... and has power over other people.'

From a psychoanalytic perspective this object which is wealthy and 'able to enjoy life to the full' harks back to the earliest period of development where the infant feels intolerable frustration as he becomes aware of the mother as separate from himself and who is seen as depriving him of the love, food and understanding that he so craves. The mother is felt to be both 'fabulously rich' and in a permanent state of satisfaction, enjoying for herself the very things of which the infant feels deprived. This pain and frustration felt in relation to this awareness is 'dealt with' by entering the object and aggressively acquiring its characteristics. The baby, through projective identification, becomes the breast/mother and believes itself to be possessed of all the admired characteristics and functions of which moments before he felt so totally bereft.

It is clear that this process is quite distinct from that described by Klein in her 1946 paper and there is a close link here to the work of Herbert Rosenfeld, who made extensive use of the concept of projective identification and elaborated it further as a result of his work with psychotic patients.

Klein's 1955 paper also gives a very clear statement of a type of projective identification which is characteristic of the depressive position. Here, projection of good parts of the self is not accompanied by depletion but on the contrary serves to enrich the ego through securing a relation between it and a world endowed with goodness.

She says: 'a securely established good object, implying a securely established love for it, gives the ego a feeling of riches and abundance which allows for an outpouring of libido and projection of good parts of the self into the external world without a sense of depletion arising' (p. 144). This bears closely on both Rosenfeld's and Bion's development of the concept but is not, however, without conceptual problems as the projective identification so described would not appear to be serving a defensive function.

Post-Kleinian developments of the concept

I will now turn to the ways in which the concept has developed, principally in the work of Herbert Rosenfeld and Wilfred Bion.

Herbert Rosenfeld was among the first psychoanalysts to treat psychotic patients using ordinary psychoanalytic technique and it was through his understanding of these patients that he was to make an important contributions to psychoanalytic theory and particularly to the theory of projective identification both by distinguishing different motives for projective identification and through a fuller discussion of the relation between projective identification and envy.

First Rosenfeld (1971b) distinguished two primary motives that underlie projective identification, communication and evacuation. Where communication is the motive, the patient wishes to make the analyst endure certain sorts of experience which the patient cannot manage or understand. 'These projective mechanisms seem to be a distortion or intensification of the normal infantile relationship' (Rosenfeld, in Spillius, 1988a, p. 121).

Example[12]

Mr K, a profoundly schizoid man arrived for his session one day and was upset to discover another patient Mr B in the waiting room. Mr B had in fact made a mistake and come at the wrong time for his session. It emerged that Mr K had felt very worried and vulnerable in this situation, and feared that his analyst would see the other patient instead of him.

In the following day's session, Mr K looked more bedraggled than usual and began his session in the following way.

'I've been to see Dr X [his previous therapist]. I get on with him. I liked him much better as a therapist than you. I am sure if I could see him three times a week, I'd make more progress than with you. I know things about him ... I don't know anything about you.'

The therapist, in discussing this session, described how he felt belittled and hurt, feeling himself to be much inferior to Dr X with whom Mr K had appeared to have a much more lively, fruitful and open relationship.

After a pause Mr K said thoughtfully, in a tentative questioning voice as if checking something, 'I don't know if that's hurtful. Is it? I don't even know if it is true.'

He went on: 'I saw this old woman in the street on the way here. I thought I could mug her or I could say hello. I wasn't sure which was best ... but I didn't put either thought into action.'

---

[12]*Note*: I am grateful to Dr Neil Morgan who discussed the following material with me.

His therapist felt touched by this and replied: 'You are trying to let me know how cast out you felt by seeing the other patient yesterday. You felt pushed into a relationship with me which you thought was second best to the one I have with the other patient, that I would rather see him than you.'

The point here is that the patient although appearing superior was also communicating (saying 'hello') to the therapist his own experience of feeling left out and vulnerable. He clearly had not lost touch with the experience and indeed seemed to be checking out if his communication had been properly registered.

The capacity of the therapist to take in the experience of feeling left out and belittled was clearly crucial to his capacity to communicate to his patient his understanding of what had taken place between them, and this suggests that the projective mechanisms facilitated the capacity for empathy.

Rosenfeld compares this more benign form of communicative projective identification with the situation where the primary aim of the process is not communication, but evacuation, namely to rid the mind of disturbing mental contents thus denying certain aspects of psychic reality. This is clearly closely related to Klein's original description of these processes. Here the subject dis-identifies himself from that which has been projected and any attempt to re-introduce such projected contents into his own mind is fiercely resisted and may even be felt as an assault. Rosenfeld makes it clear that projective identification of this sort also arises from wishes to control the object.

Example

Ms G was a patient at a stage in her analysis where the whole situation was overwhelmed by her incessant intrusive demand to possess the analyst. For example she refused to leave sessions and tried to communicate with her analyst outside session times through letters and telephone calls. In one session she seemed calmer. She talked at some length of a friend, Susan, who she thought was clearly very disturbed. Susan kept ringing her and was constantly demanding that Ms G go round to see her. She threatened suicide if Ms G did not comply with her wishes. Ms G was very angry with Susan and described her as madly possessive and greedy. Of course, when hearing this material the analyst couldn't help but be struck by how well the description of Susan fitted the patient herself. The analyst remarked to the patient that Susan seemed to represent a possessive intrusive aspect of herself. The response of the patient to this perhaps rather clumsy remark was quiet revealing. She sat bolt upright and clasped the back of her head as if she had been assaulted.

Here, then, one can see that the primary aim of the projection of aspects of herself into Susan served not communication but evacuation. The rather clumsy misdiagnosis of the situation proved to be quite traumatic to the patient. In other situations it is the analyst who is the object of these forceful projections and having to tolerate very disturbing states of mind without forcing them back into the patient becomes a central part of the analytic task.

Rosenfeld (*op. cit.*) also discusses at some length the relation between envy and projective identification. The desire to get inside the object often becomes very intense just at the point where the object is felt to be separate from the self and possessed of good and valuable qualities and thus is the target of very intense envy. One might picture this along the lines of the infant's relation with the mother. The awareness of the fact that the mother is both separate from himself and possessed of valuable qualities brings a very difficult situation, for which there are a number of possible 'solutions'. If the infant is robust enough, has built up a secure internal good object, then he is able to withstand the intense pain, a mixture of envy, frustration and pining, and so is able to retain in his mind the realistic perception of a good object that he cannot possess. This is a major developmental step. In those situations where that is not possible then the subject may project himself into the object so that he now feels himself to be possessed of its good qualities and thus awareness of separation, and the frustration that arises from this, are abolished.

Example

A young man, Mr L, believed himself to be totally self-sufficient but came into analysis when this delusion of self-sufficiency broke down. Like many patients faced with such a crisis he endeavoured to rebuild his defensive structure and tried to use the analysis to support him in that task. On a Friday session at the end of a week where there had been considerable development he gave ample evidence of his fears of feeling lonely over the weekend. When he returned for his Monday session he was elated and rather contemptuous of any suggestion that the weekend had been difficult. It had not. He had spent much of it providing for various friends, of which there seemed to be quite a number, who he felt were having a difficult time in life. Much of his looking after seemed to consist in providing them with understanding and much of this understanding, though he was quite unaware of this, was identical to that which he had gained during the previous week of analysis. This patient had dealt with the separation by becoming projectively identified with his analyst and now possessed of some of the valued qualities of his analyst he felt no feelings of separation.

In this situation described above there remains, at least at some level, a belief in the value of the analytic work, it is just that this valued function has changed psychological residence. An alternative way that this same situation can be dealt with is a source of great difficulty in analysis and of course in life. Here the subject deals with the problem not by appropriating the good object but instead by denigrating it so that it is no longer thought of as valuable. Envy here is the motive for the attack on the good object and the resulting situation also defends the subject from envy, as there is now nothing to be envious of.

Example

Miss J, a narcissistic young woman, was quite crippled by her envy of others to the extent that she found it very difficult to allow anyone to help her for, as she saw it, any person occupying such a position possessed something that she did not. At the initial stages of her analysis she would, at the beginning of session, be silent, flick her hair and look studiedly at her fingernails while I found myself becoming frustrated and impatient. I though of her as identified with a narcissistic mother preening herself while all the wishes for contact were violently projected into me, the motive here being both evacuation and control.

Some years into her analysis she, quite unusually, expressed real appreciation for an important understanding that had occurred and went on to express some regret about lost opportunities in life. Quite suddenly, as the session came near to its end, there was a dramatic change. The atmosphere became chilling and the patient said with a sneer, 'Well, if grovelling to you is what is needed [for me] to get better then that's what I'll have to do.' In this moment the patient's awareness of her good object and the inevitable pain that this brought was 'dealt with' by effecting a transformation where what might have been an awareness of a mutually satisfying relation between herself and her analyst had been, in her mind, turned into a sado-masochistic scenario where the analyst is pictured as perversely enjoying her dependence upon him.

A note on narcissism and projective identification.

The types of object relation described by Klein in 'Notes on some schizoid mechanisms' are also termed narcissistic (see Chapter 8). The massive projective processes result in the subject living in a world made up of projective aspects of himself and each new relationship soon turns into a repetition of all previous relationships. In analysis such patients tend to maintain a particular relationship with someone who remains an object of constant preoccupation. He may, for example, feel persecuted by someone at work who he feels is very envious of him. He changes jobs, yet soon sessions are again filled with accounts of someone, apparently different, at the new place of work who occupies the same position in relation to him, namely he is very envious of the patient. Although the actual identity of the person may change in these situations, the objects attributed to them do not. The 'new' person is talked about in exactly the same way as all the previous people who have occupied this position in his life. The unique qualities of the external object are obscured. As pointed out above, from the subject's point of view those aspects of himself that have been projected are distinct from himself, but from a more objective perspective one can see that the repetitiousness of his relationships arises from the fact that he is only relating to aspects of himself. Narcissus, in the myth, gazes into a pool and believes himself to be in love with another, but from our more objective position we can see that it is his own self that is the object of his fascination. As Rosenfeld (1971b) puts it:

> It will be clear that Melanie Klein gives the name 'projective identification' both to processes of ego splitting and the 'narcissistic' object relations created by projection of the self into objects. (Rosenfeld, 1971b, p. 118)

Emergence from narcissism involves a 'reclaiming' of projected aspects of the self which leads both to a new integration and brings with it the capacity to perceive the object as it really is.

Example of a patient emerging from narcissism[13]

Mr V led a very limited life marked by profound sexual inhibition. Once in his life he had a girlfriend whom he really desired but he became madly preoccupied with her and couldn't bear her being out of his sight. One of his most distressing symptoms was that if he saw strong muscular men, for example on building sites, he felt an intense urge to hug them as if to try to get inside them. At the time of the material to be reported he had a long-standing relationship with a girl who depended upon him and towards whom he felt a very hidden contempt, but he also felt very guilty about his way of treating her. He also had a constant dread of discovering that someone he felt was 'no good' was in fact more able than he. He was late for every session of his analysis.

The session to be reported was just prior to a break and followed a period of integration where he was moving away from his narcissistic attitude both in his life and in his analysis (towards which he had been very dismissive).

---

[13]*Note:* This material comes from a previous publication – see Bell and Segal (1991).

He was late for the session and, after a brief apology, went on to talk of an event that he had found very disturbing. While driving he had seen a car in his rear view mirror which from the 'configuration of the headlamps', he realized was the same model as his analyst's (it was also the same model as he himself drove for, a few weeks after starting analysis he bought a car of the same type as his analyst). He became very preoccupied with a need to know if it was his analyst's car. Some features of the car were different. He felt this preoccupation was driving him mad.

An interpretation was made along the lines that he really wanted to take a good look inside his analyst to see what sort of person he was, in particular to see if he was different from himself, something that he had previously thought unlikely.

He seemed relieved and interested in the interpretation and went on to discuss a situation he had described before, but never so vividly. He said that whenever he saw someone he believed to have certain valued qualities that he himself did not possess, he felt an immediate need to merge with or get inside this person. He called this process 'colonization'. He described the urge as unbearable. He also explained that this often happened when he suddenly saw someone he had thought 'no good' in a new light.

This material, I thinks gives a very vivid description of this patient's difficulties and of how he coped with them. Because he functioned so much through projective identification (for example, by projecting the needy aspect of himself into his girlfriend and into the analyst who always had to wait for him), his life was dull and repetitive. In the session he seemed to have been struck by the interpretation that was made, which he thought was new and which allowed him to see his analyst in a new light, as someone who was important to him. The analyst was experienced as being separate from him, not controlled by him. But this time he did not, as he often did, quickly mock the interpretation rendering it meaningless to him (i.e. an envious attack), nor did he take it over and make it his own (in the same way that he had made the analyst's car his car). He felt separate from the analyst and was immediately faced with unbearable feelings of desire for an object that he did not possess. The wish to get inside the object, through 'colonization' was a wish to wipe out the separation from the object and instead to possess it, a wish he managed to resist, at the cost of considerable pain.

The close interrelationship between projective identification and narcissism forms an important part of Rosenfeld's contribution. He also gave great emphasis to the importance of the acute mental pain caused to the patient by the confusional states that result both from projective identification and from the breakdown in the capacity to use this mechanism. This is particularly important in psychotic patients where the certainty created by projective identification is lost and the resultant doubt is felt as intolerable confusion. This was illustrated by a schizophrenic patient who agreed with the hallucinatory voices who told him his analyst was mad. However when he became a bit saner he was overwhelmed with unbearable psychic pain attendant on the recognition that, as he put it, he did 'not know anymore who was and who was not sane'.

The work of Bion

Bion made a fundamental contribution to our understanding of projective identification showing how, through subtle and complex processes, the patient manages to evoke in the object feelings that are consistent with what has been projected in fantasy. This development of the concept, which has been so extraordinarily fruitful from a clinical point of view has close links to Bion's theory of mental development (see Bion, 1962a). He suggested a model of mother–infant interaction in which the infant quite literally projects unbearable aspects of his own mind into the mother (see Chapter 12). Such a mental content might be for example the terror of annihilation. The mother's capacity to be able to receive this projection, to allow herself to be affected by it and to transform it into something manageable which is returned to the infant is, according to this account, critical for the development of the capacity to think about experience.

Through the repetition of the interactions described above the infant not only feels the relief of having various disturbing situations understood but also develops the capacity to think about his own experiences without denying them or being overwhelmed by them.

Bion, using this model, described the different types of failure that may occur in this relationship and the consequences they have for development. If the maternal 'container' is unable to take in the projections, whether this be because of the intensity of the projections, or because of deficiencies in the 'container', the consequences for development are catastrophic and the result is the severe disturbances of thinking and feeling that are characteristic of schizoid and borderline states. Such people spend much of their life evading anxiety-provoking experiences while all the time feeling persecuted by their lack of capacity to achieve this.

Bion further suggested that certain patients of this sort approach analysis to avail themselves of an opportunity that they feel they have been denied all their lives - namely to use the analyst as an object into which they can project bizarre and disturbing states of mind. In 'Attacks on linking' (1959) Bion described how the patient feels that this link, the link to the analyst afforded by projective identification, is felt to be in constant danger of being interrupted. From the patient's point of view this attack on the link with the analyst, representing the primary object, is felt to take place inside the analyst and such interruptions are felt as a terrible assault upon the patient. For some patients even the analyst's speaking or thinking is experienced as an attack upon the patient.

Example

A psychotic patient Mr F came from a very large Irish Catholic family. He had 10 siblings and each one followed within a year or so of the previous one. In analysis he conveyed a demand to be continuously understood and any failure by the analyst (which was of course frequent) resulted in states of despair and emptiness. In one session he brought a rather complex dream and conveyed an urgency that this dream be immediately understood, which the analyst was quite unable to do. When there was no immediate response the patient seemed hopeless and quite fragmented. The analyst suggested to him that when the analyst did not immediately give him the quick understanding that he so craved he experienced this as being attacked by the analyst. The patient became thoughtful again. He said that he remembered that during his breakdown he saw two newspaper headlines that he felt had great significance for him. One headline said 'There Is a Blockage On the Road' and the other said 'Colin [his name] Screams into Space'.

The patient was describing how, when he did not have available to him a link with the analyst that was immediate, he felt he was obstructed (the blockage on the road) and was left screaming out his mental contents into space. One might imagine that in such a large family, where mother was always pregnant the original blockage was felt to be the presence inside mother of another baby that stopped his having access to her.

Bion's work has focused study upon the complex ways in which patient and analyst live out together certain aspects of the patient's inner world and the understanding of these interactions has enormously enriched the understanding of the analytic task.

It is clear here that projective identification is being given a new meaning in that the actual effect upon the object, what is *really* evoked in it, begins to play a crucial part in the theory of psychoanalytic technique.

Although there has not been sufficient space here to examine them in detail our discussion of the post-Kleinian contribution to the theory of projective identification could not close without mention of three further authors. Segal (1957, 1978) elaborated the effects of projective identification on the capacity to form symbols. In the more disturbed situation the patient confuses those aspects of himself which he has projected into an object, with the object itself. In these situations the symbol is confused with the thing symbolized and Segal described the result as a 'symbolic equation', quite distinct from true symbolism which can only occur when there is separation from the object (see Chapter 10). Meltzer (1966) has made a very important contribution in our understanding of the types of confusion that result from projective identification where there is a confusion of bodily zones. Sohn (1985) has brought a very useful conceptual clarification, through his description of what he terms 'the identificate' formed when part of the ego, through projecting itself into an object, acquires an omnipotence which forms the core of a narcissistic organization. He emphasizes the stability of this structure and like Rosenfeld sees it as being both an expression of envy and serving to abolish awareness of envy, vulnerability and dependence. Unlike Rosenfeld he does not think that introjective identification has any major role to play in these situations.

Conclusion

In this chapter I have reviewed the history of the concept of projective identification from its origins to the present day. It will be clear that the term covers a number of different processes. One thorny issue arises from consideration of the significance of the effect upon the external object. Here there appear to be two positions. Some have suggested, and this is particularly so in the American school, that the capacity to evoke feelings in the object enters into the definition of projective identification. From this point of view, if the analyst is not affected then the mechanism is not projective identification. There is I think a difficulty here, as such an account would appear to create some confusion through the conflation of a mental mechanism and a clinical experience both of which occupy different conceptual domains.

The point of view presented in this chapter is rather different. Projective identification corresponds to an unconscious phantasy where aspects of the self can be located in other objects. This phantasy has real effects upon the mind of the subject who then behaves as if, for example, he *really is* rid of some unwanted part of himself, and this is so, I would suggest, regardless of the effect upon the object. When the object is provoked into feeling the state of mind which the projector has projected then I think it is better to regard this not as projective identification per se but as the actualization (Sandler, 1976a, 1976b) of the unconscious phantasy. The ways in which these phantasies can become actualized has become a very important area of contemporary psychoanalytic research (see for example Joseph, 1989; Feldman, 1997).

Most Kleinian authors would I think agree that the effect upon the object is not a necessary condition that *enters into the definition* of projective identification but many would, I think, follow Spillius (1988a) in suggesting that it is helpful to distinguish those situations where the projective identification evokes the appropriate feeling state in the object from those where it does not.

I will end this chapter therefore with a classification of projective identification (Figure 9.1) that makes use of the distinctions drawn by Rosenfeld, Spillius and Britton, referred to above.

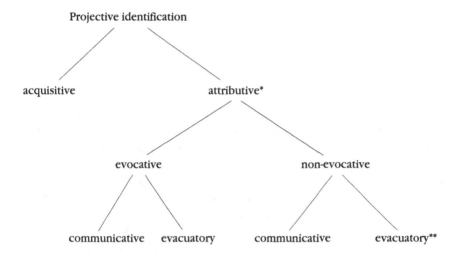

*It should be noted that acquisitive and attributive projective identification, although separated here for clasification, usually happen together
** This category may seem strange in that it might be thought that a projective identification that does not evoke any response in the object could not be communicative. This is one of the problems of attempting a classification! But perhaps it is possible for there to be situations where no response is evoked in an external object but the projector remains psychically in touch with what he has projected and in that sense remains in communication with it.

Figure 9.1 Classification of projective identification.

CHAPTER 10

Symbolization

HANNA SEGAL

The concept of unconscious symbolism is basic and crucial in psychoanalytical theory and practice. The understanding of unconscious symbolism is the key, not only to the understanding of dreams and symptoms, but to all unconscious communication. We come to know the unconscious by its symbolic expression. It was Freud's understanding that a hysterical symptom has a meaning in that it represents something of which the patient is not conscious – that was the key opening the door to the world of the unconscious. But for many years that monumental discovery was, in a way, taken for granted. It was used as a tool for interpretation and clinical work but symbolism as such was not investigated much.

In 1916, partly pressed by the necessity to differentiate the psychoanalytical view of symbolism from that of Jung, Jones (1916) wrote his major paper on symbolism. In it he defined what he called true unconscious symbolism in the following way:

(i) A symbol represents what has been repressed from consciousness, and the whole process of symbolization is carried on unconsciously.

(ii) All symbols represent ideas of 'the self and of immediate blood relatives, or of the phenomena of birth, love and death'.

(iii) A symbol has a constant meaning. Many symbols can be used to represent the same repressed idea, but a given symbol has a constant meaning which is universal.

(iv) Symbolism arises as the result of intrapsychic conflict between the 'repressing tendencies and the repressed'. Further: 'Only what is repressed is symbolized; only what is repressed needs to be symbolized.'

Jones further distinguishes between sublimation and symbolization. 'Symbols', he says, 'arise when the affect investing the symbolized idea has not, as far as the symbol is concerned, proved capable of that modification in quality which is denoted by the term sublimation.'

148

Summarizing Jones' points, one might say that when a desire has to be given up because of conflict and repressed, it may express itself in a symbolical way, and the object of the desire which had to be given up can be replaced by a symbol.

Of the points he states, some remain uncontroversial. For instance, that the whole process is carried out unconsciously and that symbols represent the self, the immediate objects of desire and their relationships, and also, that symbolism is the result of intrapsychic conflicts. Other points have since been opened to controversy. For instance, is it really so that a symbol symbolizes only one thing? Are not symbols over-determined? Take, for instance, the snake. It symbolizes the penis; also often the faecal penis, the poisonous nipple, or even the baby's poisonous mouth. Sometimes it symbolizes all these things, and is over-determined. It also symbolizes wisdom (the snake of Hippocrates). Defining symbols as an alternative to sublimation is also open to doubt. In fact, in practice, both Freud and Jones analysed the symbolism of works of art. Melanie Klein, in contradistinction to Jones, considered that all sublimation depends on symbolism.

In one of her first papers, 'The role of the school in the Libidinal development of the child', Melanie Klein describes what school and schoolwork symbolize to the child (Klein, 1923b). Often the school represents the mother's body, with the teacher as a father; or a part object, penis, inside the mother's body. The child's school activities, play or learning, symbolize unconscious processes. Even individual letters can carry a symbolic meaning. She speaks of a little boy who could never put together the letters 'I' and 'E', because to him putting the letters together represented intercourse. Probably at the time, Klein was not even very aware that her view was departing from Freud's. Those differences were rooted in the way she looked at unconscious phantasy which was different from Freud's way. For her, unconscious phantasy was always active and ubiquitous in the child's life, and expressing itself symbolically in all activities, not only pathological symbols (see Chapter 2).

Working with children, she was unavoidably drawn into the study of the development of speech, intellectual functions, interest in the world, as well as the pathology of this development. In her view, symbolism arises from the conflict that the child experiences in relation to his mother's body. His libidinal and aggressive interest in his mother's, and later in both his parents' bodies, leads to anxiety and guilt which force him to displace his interest to the world around him, thus endowing it with symbolic meaning.

While Freud and Jones considered that it is the libidinal link which allows the child to symbolize his own and the parents' bodies by objects in the external world, Melanie Klein added the role played by anxiety as a major spur in symbol-formation. In the psychotic, symbol-formation is at its most disturbed, and it is the analysis of a psychotic child, the first of its kind, that enabled her to describe and analyse a disturbance of symbol-formation. I am referring here to her paper 'The importance of symbol-formation in the development of the ego' (Klein, 1930). In that paper, she describes the analysis of an autistic child. As it appeared in the analysis, Dick made in phantasy a very sadistic attack on his mother's body, projecting into her his excreta and parts of his body, which then became identified with parts of her. As a result of these attacks, his mother's body became an object of such intense anxiety that the whole process came to a stop. As, during the analysis, the unconscious anxiety diminished and became more manifest, the process of symbol-formation was set again in motion, enabling the child to speak, play and establish relationships. Melanie Klein came to the conclusion that anxiety spurs the development of symbolism, but excessive anxiety may paralyse it.

Klein's work was a big step in the thinking about symbolism. It related its development to that of object-relationships, and addressed itself to the pathology in that area (see Chapter 8). But it did not by itself illuminate some of its mysteries. For instance, Freud has stated that every man marries his mother. And yet, when he was told that a colleague married a much older woman he expostulated 'How could he marry a woman old enough to be his mother?' In both cases, the wife is the symbol of the mother. But what is the difference? This problem became open to investigation only with Klein's concepts of the paranoid-schizoid position and projective identification (see Chapters 3 and 9). It seems to me that Dick's attacks on his mother's body were by projective identification – one of the clearest examples, and yet pre-dating by many years, Mrs Klein's theoretical conceptualization of projective identification.

I have tried to put symbol-formation and its vicissitudes in relation to the newer concepts. I was particularly interested in trying to sort out the differentiation of symbolism in symptom-formation and in sublimation. In my paper, 'Notes on symbol formation' (Segal 1957), I gave the following example:

A patient in mental hospital says he cannot play the violin because he will not masturbate in public. Another patient plays the violin and his material makes it clear that to him, too, the violin represents the penis.

What is the difference in the symbolism? In my paper, I made the suggestion that symbol-formation develops gradually from paranoid-schizoid to a depressive level of functioning. When symbols are formed by projective identification, the result is what I called a symbolic equation. A part of the ego becomes identified with the object and, as a consequence, the symbol is equated with the thing symbolized. The symbol does not represent the object, but is treated as though it was the object. Playing the violin is felt to be masturbation. A 16-year old hebephrenic patient of mine used to bite her way through my volumes of *The Arabian Nights*. When she was sane she was an avid reader. In the depressive position, the object is given up and mourned, and the symbol is set up in the inner world – an internal object to begin with, representing the object, but not to be equated with it. The symbolic equation is used to deny the separateness between the subject and the object. The symbol is used to overcome an accepted loss. At moments of regression, symbolism may revert to a concrete form. As a child, my hebephrenic patient used to write stories about the Lancashire witches. Subsequently, she had hallucinations and delusions about the Lancashire witches pursuing her. In the sessions there were constant fluctuations between being able to tell me a phantasy or experiencing it as an hallucination or delusion about me. This happens not only in psychotics.

For instance, Mr R, a borderline patient of mine, had occasional hallucinations though he never quite believed them and kept telling himself 'that is my fabrication'. One day he came to the session terribly upset because he had had an hallucination in the morning of a little motorcyclist with a sort of helmet driving right into his head. He felt he would burst his head and it would drive him mad. Then he told himself 'it cannot be real – it must be an hallucination – my own fabrication' and the hallucination disappeared. But he looked at his index finger and suddenly realized that his index finger looked exactly like the helmet of the motorcyclist which also looked like the head of a gorilla. His association to the gorilla was that he saw a psychotic adolescent with a malformed head and he associated his finger with anal masturbation. We had recently been analysing his anal masturbation and the phantasy that was associated with it which was a violent anal penetration into the body and mind of the analyst/mother. Thus it became clear that the motorcyclist represented his own masturbating index finger projected into the motorcyclist coming back at him. (He had heard a motorcycle outside the consulting room the day before.) So, in a patient generally capable of symbolizing there were moments of regression – a very primitive pathological projective identification resulting in concrete experiences.

I shall use some sessions from later on in R's analysis to show interlinking of the development of symbolism in the Oedipal situation.

One day, he told me that, as he was going past my consulting-room door to the waiting-room, he became very anxious because the thought occurred to him that there was no guard at the door and nothing to stop him from getting into the consulting-room and interfering with the session of my other patient. Then he added, 'Come to think of it, there is nothing to stop me doing what I want on the couch. For instance, if I wanted to, I could lie upside-down.' Then he giggled and became embarrassed as he realized that upside-down in the bed is the position he was in during some love-play with his girlfriend the night before. So apparently the situation was as follows: There is no guard at the door, no husband. He could have intercourse with me as his girlfriend and have our positions upside-down; that is, with him dominating me – apparently a plain Oedipal situation. He went on to tell me a dream. He said:

> I had a dream in which I was explaining to M [the girlfriend] about my hallucina-
> tions. I was telling her, 'Look, I dream up a car, and there it is.' And the car
> appears. He got into the front seat. But there was no partition between front and
> back - no pole to lean against. He started falling backward, feeling an utmost
> panic.

And he woke up with severe anxiety.

My understanding of his associations preceding the telling of the dream, and the dream was as follows. The pole is a phallic symbol. But also I am of Polish origin, and he knew that my husband's name was Paul. In the absence of the pole, the father, or the penis in the vagina, there is nothing to stop him, not just from having intercourse with his mother on a genital level, there is nothing to stop him from unrestrained projective identification with her, and what should be an awareness of his thoughts is experienced as an external fact – something happening in mother's body. The car he dreamt of appears as an external fact. What used to be his thoughts (what he 'dreamed up') is felt by him as a reality in the external world. But the whole process, instead of an hallucination, at that point gave rise to a dream. Some time later in his analysis, it became apparent that his hallucinations disappeared from the time this dream had been analysed.

Several years later, after considerable change and improvement, the patient was getting married. Before his wedding, for which he was missing a few days of his analysis, he showed considerable ambivalence towards me, repre-senting the father. When he came back from his honeymoon he said that he had never been so moved in his life as he was at the actual wedding ceremony. He had decided to marry in church in deference to his dead father, though he himself was not religious. He had asked for his father's favourite hymn – 'The Lord's My Shepherd' – to be sung at the wedding ceremony. He said that he had never in his life been so happy and so unhappy at one and the same time. He did not know if at that moment he was regaining his father or losing him. He was so aware of his father's presence in his thoughts, and so acutely aware of his real absence from the wedding. He then told me a dream he had had the night before, in which a fisherman was to take him out to teach him fishing. The fisherman's hands were bandaged because they had cuts on them. But the fisherman assured him that he could still keep his promise.

In the last session before the break, I had occasion to point out to him that he was very cutting to me. I was the fisherman/father with the bandaged hand, but one who was not so resentful as to withdraw his help.

One can see that the first dream is what I would call pseudo-Oedipal. On the face of it, his first associations to that dream are of an Oedipal nature, wanting to make love to the mother/analyst. But what the dream reveals is something quite different. What he wants is to project himself into the analyst in a way which results in confusion and panic. In the second dream, on the contrary, the father is seen as a separate person, with a truly Oedipal ambivalence, the experience of loss and guilt. This can lead to an introjection and a positive identification with his father's masculine qualities.

There is also a difference in his mental functioning. The first dream explains his propensity to hallucinate, a failure of adequate symbolization – what he thinks *is*. In the second dream the external and the internal situations are clearly distinguished. He is aware of his father's real absence, since he is dead; and at the same time his presence in his own mind. His thought is not an hallucination but a memory of experience. And he experiences true depressive mourning. This material also illustrates the importance of the role of the father in the resolution of the Oedipus Complex and particularly his role as an object separate from mother and one which puts a stop to what could be an endless mutual projective identification between the infant and his mother.

Klein has related the troubles of symbol formation to excessive sadism. I related them to the excessive use of projective identification. Bion took the next step. In his 1957 paper he differentiated between neurotic and psychotic parts of the personality (Bion, 1957a). He stated that the difference was qualitative rather than quantitative. In his view projective identification in the psychotic process is different in kind from more benign forms of projective identification. In pathological projective identification part of the ego is mentally fragmented and projected into an object which becomes equally fragmented and identified with the projected bits. This results in the creation of what he calls bizarre objects which are minute fragments of the ego embodied and identified with parts of the object and imbued with hostility. When this happens, the mind, instead of having thoughts and symbols, is filled with bizarre objects. A patient of mine had an hallucination of thousands of computers invading his brain. Previously he had had plans of installing computers in all the schools of England so that his teaching would predominate and control the schools. The hallucinated computers were the returning bizarre objects which he projected into the world. He also associated to the thousands of interpretations which invaded his brain and were lodged in it. We were familiar from the past with his constant attempts to invade, control and disintegrate my mind and my interpretations at times of his breakdown were often felt by him to be the return of bizarre objects. The analysis of this process in the transference resolved the hallucination in that session (see Chapter 13). One could look at the hallucination of the non-psychotic Mr R also as a return of a bizarre object.

Bion extended his work in that area to his theory of the container and contained and the transformation of beta elements – those elements of concrete symbolization – and alpha elements which become elements of symbolization and thinking (Bion, 1962a).

In recent years, we have been paying increasing attention to the relationship between the early Oedipal situation, and processes of symbolization and thinking. I have contended that adequate symbolization can be established only with the working-through of the depressive position and the differentiation between external and internal realities. I have become increasingly convinced that accepting the reality of the father and the Oedipal couple is essential in this process. Attacks on the parental couple, and the links between the parents, unavoidably disrupt processes of thinking. Hatred of the parental coupling becomes a hatred of thinking. Britton describes a patient who, whenever she thought he was thoughtful, would scream at him 'Stop this fucking thinking!' (Britton, 1989, p. 88).

Bion's work on the container and contained shows how through alpha function, beta elements are transformed into alpha elements (see Chapter 12). He mostly presents this as a two-body relationship. He occasionally mentioned a third body but he does not connect it explicitly with the beginnings of an Oedipal situation. Britton extended this model, linking it with the inclusion of a third object, and extending the idea of a container to a triangular situation (Britton, 1989). He describes it as a triangle with three apexes: Father, Mother and Child. The lines between the apexes would represent the various relationships: Child–Mother, Child–Father and Father–Mother. Whereas the container–contained relationship between mother and child is wholly beneficial to the child, if things go well, that which includes father is more complicated, because it always includes a third excluded, or rather a third aware, observing the other two. That third excluded can be seen as either hostile and disruptive to the other two, in which case the mother-and-child containment is disrupted, or it can be seen as benevolent or as objective observer. This objective observer becomes that part of the child mind capable of observing the reality, and thinking about it. This seems to be a very complex and abstract concept, the triangular container. And yet, when one knows about it, it can be clinically very vivid. To give but one example:

Mrs D was tormented by recurring panics. Though intelligent, when in a state of panic, whether conscious or unconscious, she loses her concentration and all ability to think. In one of the sessions, she described acute anxieties about a hole in a wall. Some building work had to be done in her house. She could not imagine it being done without a big hole in the wall. She thought her children could fall through the hole, or herself, and anyway the thought of this big black hole triggered a sense of panic. It was fairly clear in the session that she had no idea in her mind that the builder might know what he was doing. (The transference implications were obvious.) When this was interpreted she told me that she had another panic which assailed her on the way to the session. She had lost her diary, which had confidential information about herself and the work in her office, involving other people, and the loss of the diary could be catastrophic. It slowly emerged that the loss of the diary had to do with her having read a poster of a lecture I was giving, jointly with a man. She did not intend to attend this event, but she also wanted to forget the date, not to be troubled by it. The indiscretion referred to what she felt was the indecency of my exhibiting myself on a platform with the man.

The next session was very difficult, and analytic work was hardly possible because of the patient's determination to break any links. Two themes seem to have emerged. The first one was related to an internal tormentor. It eventually led to a phantasy of a hand cruelly squeezing out a breast that was filled with a boil. The second theme referred to sexuality. She felt that I and others were trying to impose on her a view of sexual intercourse as something pleasurable and non-destructive, which was a denial, an idealization, since 'I thought everybody knew that sex was always sado-masochistic.' Another view she had of sex was as of two people coming together in intercourse in cruelty to the third person, in front of whom they were exhibiting, so as to inflict on this third person unbearable feelings of exclusion, inferiority and jealousy. Some links could be established, for instance, the parents/myself cruelly exhibiting to the child and the resulting destruction of her relationship to the breast; but the patient remained on the whole disconnected from me, angry, and very anxious.

In the third session, as she was speaking of the hole, some music from the neighbouring flat could just be heard in the consulting-room. She drew my attention to it, and said it made her think of people dancing. She did not feel disturbed or persecuted by it. Eventually we could establish that the terrible hole in her mind was the missing space in which she could perceive the parents, represented by me, dancing together. Later in the session, she started speaking about her difficulties in writing a report she had to do at work, but in a much quieter and understanding way. This patient had an idealizing relationship to the breast, but this relationship was very fragile, only to be maintained by a splitting-off of ambivalence. The appearance of a third object turned everything into torment. Not only was she tormented by phantasies of sexuality infused with cruelty, but also the original relation to the breast was destroyed by this intrusion and also turned into torment. When this intrusion happened, her mind became itself disjointed and fragmented, and she became filled with intense paranoid and hypochondriacal phantasies. At those points her capacity for understanding and symbolization got lost. My talking to others was experienced as my forcing her to witness an actual sexual intercourse. The bad feelings about me became a tormented and tormenting poisonous breast inside her, experienced in her physical symptoms. She could get rid of the resulting persecution by making a hole in her mind instead of a space accommodating the dancing parents, though later in the third session she showed how the containment and understanding provided by the analytic situation led to a transformation of beta into alpha elements.

In this Chapter I have tried to show that symbolism is a continuous evolving process from the beginning of mental life. It is central in all our mental activities. One could define man as an animal capable of symbolization. What do we mean when we say 'x is in touch with his unconscious?' Obviously, we do not mean that he is consciously aware, for instance, of cannibalistic phantasies, etc. What we do mean is that he is in touch with their symbolic representation. Thus symbolism is crucial in internal communication between parts of ourselves. It is of course also and more evidently essential in communication with others, non-verbal as well as verbal. Thus it is that clinically we are confronted with problems of symbolization and its peripatetics, most immediately and directly in psychotics because of the failure to communicate, and in artists because their life is centred on symbolization, using universal symbols in new ways and creating new symbols.

CHAPTER 11

Changing models of the mind

HANNA SEGAL

Almost from the beginning, when formulating a theory of mind, Freud saw the mind as having a structure. I think it is not often appreciated or emphasized how revolutionary that way of looking at the mind was. Until Freud, the mind was a rather vague concept. Seeing it as a structure implied that the psychic world, like the physical world, can be studied in terms of elements, or parts, combining into a structure. This can become a subject of detailed study of the different parts and their interactions.

I said that the various elements, or parts, combine to form a structure, because it is an important aspect of Freud's theory that structures are also seen by him in dynamic terms. They are the result of dynamic conflicting forces; not only forces in the past, defining a structure once and for all; he also saw it as something happening in the present, that is, that the same forces which were responsible for setting up the structure continue to maintain it. The implication of this is that if the interplay of those forces changes, there is a possibility of a change in the structure, and this of course, is essential from the point of view of therapeutic possibilities. One of the earliest of Freud's statements about the therapeutic aims was 'Where id was there ego shall be' (Freud, 1933a, p. 80). This is at least a quantitative, if not a qualitative, change in the structure.

Freud's first model of the mind, known as the topographical model, is also structural, since it describes the structure of the mind in three layers – Conscious, Preconscious and Unconscious. It is also dynamic. It is the forces of repression that keep the id unconscious. The preconscious Freud originally thought of as containing those elements which are not at the moment conscious, but are readily available to consciousness. However, the later concept included the idea of a censor between the Preconscious and Conscious, where there was a conflict, and dynamic elements in maintaining or releasing the censorship. In Freud's later structural model of the mind the id is roughly equated to what had previously been contained by the concept of the Unconscious, the superego becomes an agency that carries the 'functions which have hitherto been performed by the people [the abandoned objects] in the external world: it observes the ego, gives it orders, judges it and threatens it with punishments, exactly like the parents whose place it has taken' (Freud, 1938, p. 205) while the ego becomes an agency of the mental apparatus in conflict with 'Its three tyrannical masters ... the external world, the superego and the id' (Freud, 1933a, p. 77).

What is known as the structural theory of mind, though not contradicting and excluding the topographical description, introduces new and most important elements. I think it is the structural theory on which most modern psychoanalysis is based.

As this work developed, Freud introduced important modifications to his theory of instincts, anxiety, and mental structure. In the 1920s, he reformulated some of his basic ideas. Originally he thought that the basic conflict was between the libido and the self-preservative instinct, more linked with the reality-sense. By 1920, in *Beyond the Pleasure Principle*, he put forward his new and last theory of instincts. He saw the basic conflict as being between the life instinct and the death instinct, and the libido as part of the life instinct in conflict with the death instinct, which, turned outwards, became aggression (Freud, 1920a).

The new element that Freud introduced into his view of the structure is the essential role of an internal object relationship (see Chapter 8). There is the ego and the id, as in the previous model; but a crucial role is played by an internal object – the superego. Concurrently and inevitably the mechanism of introjection becomes central; an internal object is a parental (in Freud's original view, paternal) object that has been actively introjected. But this introjected object is one that is also filled with projections. In Freud's well-known diagram of the pyramid in *The Ego and the Id* (Freud, 1923), the base is the id, but the superego is filled with the id. Freud originally explained this in complex ways to do with cathexis and de-cathexis; but in some later papers he attributed this phenomenon to projections into the superego. Freud's new and last theory of instincts also affects this model. In *The Ego and the Id* he speaks of the superego of the melancholic being a 'pure culture of the death instinct' (Freud, 1923, p. 53).

One of my first patients in the first week of his analysis had the following dream:

The patient, who was a naval officer, and had no previous knowledge of psychoanalysis, dreamt of a pyramid. *At the bottom of this pyramid there was a group of rough sailors bearing a gold book on their heads. On this book stood a naval officer of the same rank as himself, and on his shoulders stood an admiral. The admiral, the patient said, seemed in his own*

way to exercise as great a pressure from above, and to be as awe-inspiring
as the group of sailors who formed the base of the pyramid and pressed
from below.

Having told me this dream, he said, 'This is myself. This is my world. The
gold book represents a golden mean, a road on which I tried to keep. I am
squashed between the pressure of my instincts and what I want to do, and
the prohibitions coming to me from my conscience.' He had some associations to his current situation, where as a second officer he had to negotiate
between the captain of the ship and a rather unruly crew. He also associated
how he felt squashed by his father when he was a child; though he felt that in
reality his father was not nearly as awesome as the figure in the dream. This
dream seemed to illustrate his inner world almost with the accuracy of
Freud's diagram.

Klein's work extends Freud's model. It is not that the superego disappears
from her formulation. But it is, as it were, put under the microscope. And she
investigates the forces that give it its character. Though Klein took as her
basis Freud's theory of instincts, and particularly the conflict between the life
and death instincts, I think she refers less and less frequently to the concept
of the id as a separate part of the personality. If she were here she might not
agree with me; but my own view of the Kleinian model does not actually
include the id as a structure. I view it more as the ego, being the I, which has
perceptions, instincts and desires, which express themselves in object
relationships. The structure of the ego is determined by the way the ego
organizes its object-relationships, which in phantasy it internalizes and makes
part of itself. The relation of structure and function is reciprocal. It is the
function that determines the structure but the structure in turn affects the
function. For instance, the over-severe superego increases anxiety and
mobilizes defensive manoeuvres in the ego.

Freud has said that the ego is a precipitate of abandoned object-cathexis
(Freud, 1933a, p. 77). This formulation came before he described the
superego, a concept which he introduced later. One could assume that this
precipitate is the superego. However, I think that there are two aspects of
that precipitate: while some introjects are maintained as separate objects,
with which the ego has a relationship – the superego described by Freud –
other aspects of the object are introjected into the ego, and the ego identifies
with them. If ego-syntonic, they contribute to the ego's growth. In the structural model, the ego is not identified with consciousness, but much of it is
unconscious.

Freud dated the introjection of the father as a superego to the resolution
of the Oedipus Complex. Klein traces the superego to its primitive roots. She
extends the concept of phantasy (see Chapter 2). In her view the relation to
the object and phantasy exist from birth, and from the beginning there are

active processes of splitting, projection and introjection. And she provides her own model of the structure. She describes two different potential positions of the ego and its internal objects: one is what she called the paranoid-schizoid position (see Chapter 3), in which the object is split between an ideal and a persecutory one, the roots of the ego-ideal and the persecutory superego. It is filled with projections and often fragmented. Parallel with this – and Klein paid particular attention to this state of the ego (though hers is not called Ego Psychology) – the ego is split between what is held to be its good and its bad parts, and also frequently fragmented. Klein saw the evolution of the structure in terms of withdrawal of projections, lessening of fragmentation, lessening of splits, restructuring the ego and its objects, from split to whole: in other words, what she named the depressive position (see Chapter 4).

To return to my patient who dreamt of the pyramid. As his analysis progressed, it became clear that the model he presented of his mind was based on a deep split. His association 'This is my world' referred also to the fact that the dream contained only men, and, similarly, his life seemed to be spent with men. It is not an accident that he joined the Navy. When he spoke of his 'instincts' he was referring to his strong homosexual impulses and phantasies, which he had to keep completely suppressed while on the ship. He was an extremely conscientious and 'proper' officer. Split off from this, he had an intensely idealized phantasy of an idealized and asexual mother, and one he identified with – becoming extremely caring and protective, and trying hard to be completely asexual in relation to young sailors. All his hatred and eroticism were displaced onto his relation with his father. As his splits and projections were identified, he had to face an acute conflict of ambivalence in relation to his mother and to the parents as a couple, and also to face acute depressive feelings.

This in itself does not conflict with Freud's id-ego-superego model. Nevertheless, there is a shift of emphasis to the importance of object-relationships. It is the way the ego in phantasy organizes its objects which determines the structure. In Klein's view, splitting, fragmentation and projection belong to the paranoid-schizoid position, and it is only in the depressive position, with the awareness of ambivalence and guilt, that repression sets in. But there is a complication in this model, in the sense that the evolution is never completed, and in fact both positions co-exist, and there is a fluctuation between them. The depressive position is characterized by intense psychic pain, and this pain leads to repeated regressions to the paranoid-schizoid position (see Chapter 4).

Is it then that the mind has two structures? Or is it that the one evolves into the other? In a way both statements are true. There is an evolution that is never completed, and the paramount question in relation to mental life is:

which one is the central core of the personality? And if the structure is the more mature structure of the depressive position, how much is this central core under threat from more archaic structures? I think Bion's work is helpful in further elucidating this problem. He proposes a different view of the model. In fact, in some of his writings he speaks of a new metapsychology. His model has as its central position the relationship between the container and the contained (see Chapter 12).

Bion extends Klein's concept of projective identification into a model in which the infant projects beta elements into the maternal breast where they undergo a transformation into alpha elements. Beta elements are inchoate sense data, including emotional data experienced concretely, they 'are not felt to be phenomena, but things in themselves' (Bion, 1962a, p. 6). Alpha elements are elements of feeling, thinking, and phantasy. The infant projects beta elements into the mother. If the mother is receptive to these projections, her understanding – her own alpha function – transforms them into alpha. When this container–contained conjunction is internalized it becomes what Bion calls the mental apparatus. But one could see it also as a basic structuring of the ego. And he makes it clear that the formation of this apparatus is coexistent with the shift from the paranoid-schizoid to depressive functioning. Melanie Klein, among other things, contended that in the shift between the paranoid-schizoid and depressive position repression takes over from splitting as the leading mechanism.

Bion amplifies that statement, and looks from another angle at what is meant by repression. He looks on repression as a contact barrier, not a caesura, but a part of the mind, in which there is a constant on-going transformation between the beta and alpha elements (Bion, 1962a, p. 26). In that barrier, processes of symbolization happen which allow primitive contents to be transformed and used by the ego, allowing the person continuous contact with his or her unconscious, in a way necessary to be in contact with external reality as well. This amplifies the idea about repression I formulated in my work on symbolism (see Chapter 10), when I suggested that what Freud called excessive repression was in fact a splitting-off of insufficiently symbolized material, whereas more normal repression gives rise to symbolization and further elaboration. One could view the contact barrier described by Bion as enabling a constant transformation, in Freud's terminology, of the id into the ego; in Klein's, from paranoid-schizoid to depressive functioning; and in his own terminology, from beta to alpha. When this process fails, a beta screen gets formed – a cluster of beta elements.

Bion also suggests that the contact barrier can be seen both as a function and as a structure in the mind. This is also consistent with the topographical model, but it is much more dynamic, and more fluid. In his view, every significant event is at depth experienced as a beta element which gets transformed into alpha: a constant ongoing process of transformation from the most primitive contents to beta, to alpha, to symbolization, and eventually into preconscious verbalization. This evolution, however, involves psychic pain at all its points: feelings of separateness, depressive guilt, Oedipal pain; so at any stage this process can be impeded. And when it is impeded, pathological structures are formed, pathological organization, as described by John Steiner (1993, p. 4). And this has important clinical implications. I think we direct our attention primarily to the point at which pathological structures are born. This could be seen as a new look at Freud's concept of fixation points.

I am well aware that there are other views of the evolution of mental structure, for instance the Kohutian, but to my mind these are often less consistent with Freud's original model. I have confined myself to the Freud–Klein–Bion models which are familiar to me and which I find compatible and useful.

It is a claim of psychoanalysis that psychoanalytic treatment, in contrast to other therapies, does effect structural changes. The change in our view of the structure of the mind must be unavoidably linked with changes in our view of therapeutic factors of psychoanalysis, and have an influence on technique, while, conversely, it is of course changes in technique that often lead to new discoveries and changes in our theoretical views.

As I have tried to show, the mental structure evolves from the most primitive to the more mature levels. What militates against this evolution? Freud spoke of fixation points at various libidinal stages. I think we still think, though in a different way, of something like fixation points – points at which this evolution is interfered with. The therapeutic aim is to address those points and allow normal evolution to proceed (see Chapter 13).

Money-Kyrle, in a speech given at his eightieth birthday, described the evolution of his views. He considered that when he was in his analysis with Freud, he thought that pathology was due to the repression of the libido. In his second analysis, with Klein, he understood that pathology was rooted in a conflict between the destructive and libidinal impulses. Later on, he came to believe that the pathology was mainly based on a misperception (linked with original pathological projective identification).

These statements, I think, correspond closely to evolution in our thinking in his long psychoanalytic lifetime. Freud's first idea was that pathology was due to excessive repression, and the psychoanalytic work consisted in lifting repressions: 'Where id was ego shall be.' The ego regains mastery of the id by insight and understanding. I think that in psychoanalytic thinking the importance of insight remains crucial. But this is not the same as dealing simply with repression. When Freud reviewed his views of the model of the mind, and introduced the importance of the superego it became clear that factors other than simple repression were at work. For instance, diminishing the severity of the nature of the superego became a major concern.

Strachey, in his major paper, 'The nature of the therapeutic action of psychoanalysis' (1934), addressed this issue. He bases his work on Freud's new model, presented in *The Ego and the Id*, and addresses himself to the fate of the superego in the psychoanalytic process. How is it that the superego is arrested at the primitive level? He uses Klein's new discoveries (preceding her final formulation) of the paranoid-schizoid and depressive position.

I will re-state what I believe to be her views in an exceedingly schematic outline. The individual, she holds, is perpetually introjecting and projecting into the objects of its id-impulses, and the character of the introjected objects depends on the character of the id-impulses directed towards the external objects. Thus, for instance, during the stage of a child's libidinal development in which it is dominated by feelings of oral aggression, his feelings towards the external object will be orally aggressive; he will then introject the object, and the introjected object will now act (in the manner of the superego) in an orally aggressive way towards the child's ego. The next event will be the projection of this orally aggressive introjected object back on to the external object, which will now in its turn appear to be orally aggressive. The fact of the external object being thus felt as dangerous and destructive once more causes the id-impulses to adopt an even more aggressive and destructive attitude towards the object in self-defence. A vicious circle is thus established. This process seeks to account for the extreme severity of the superego in small children, as well as for their unreasonable fear of outside objects. In the course of the development of the normal individual, his libido eventually reaches the genital stage, at which the positive impulses predominate. His attitude towards his external objects will thus become more friendly, and accordingly his introjected object (or superego) will become less severe and his ego's contact with reality will be less distorted. In the case of the neurotic however, for various reasons – whether on account of frustration or of an incapacity of the ego to tolerate id-impulses, or of an inherent excess of the destructive components – development to the genital stages does not occur, but the individual remains fixated at a pre-genital level. His ego is thus left exposed to the pressure of a savage id on the one hand and a correspondingly savage superego on the other, and the vicious circle I have just described is perpetuated.

I should like to suggest that the hypothesis which I have stated in this bald fashion may be useful in helping us to form a picture not only of the mechanism of a *neurosis* but also of the mechanism of its *cure*. There is, after all, nothing new in regarding a neurosis as essentially an obstacle or deflecting force in the path of normal development; nor is there anything new in the belief that psychoanalysis, owing to the peculiarities of the analytic situation, is able to remove the obstacle and so allow the normal development to proceed.

Strachey emphasizes the role of unconscious phantasy, primitive object-relationships, and the importance of projection and introjection. And he introduces the concept of a mutative interpretation: in his view, the mutative interpretation is that interpretation of the transference, which changes the very nature of the superego. In his view of the psychoanalytic process, the patient projects his archaic superego into the analyst and reintrojects it, modified by the analyst's understanding. In that way, the archaic severity of the superego is modified and the reality ego is strengthened. He makes it quite clear that this does not mean that the analyst should act like a 'good object'. This would only reinforce the split between the idealized and the persecutory superego. It is the analyst's capacity to contain the bad projections, and understand them, which leads to the integration between the idealized and the persecutory figure.

Further work of Klein, and later her followers, added something to Strachey's model. The work on projective identification showed that it is not only an internal object or objects that are projected into the analyst, but parts of the patient's own ego (see Chapter 9). The problem is not only a distorted view of the object but also of severe losses to the ego. Very importantly among them, the ego's capacity to form judgments may be projected in the process. This further work also brought to the fore the importance of the levels of communication. This is blatant in psychosis, in which the patient's communication is on the level of concrete thinking: thoughts and feelings are replaced by misperceptions, hallucinations, actions, etc; and the analyst's task is to trace these to the projections which lead to psychotic functioning.

Bion's model extends that of Strachey and Klein to include the most primitive levels. The analyst's function is to contain beta projections, and this understanding converts beta into alpha elements. As I see it, the alpha function gives beta elements psychic meaning. Disturbances of these processes are blatant, as I have said, in the psychotic; but they also underlie neurotic symptomatology, where the psychotic process is encapsulated in an area of psychotic functioning. For instance, in crowd phobia the crowd is at depth experienced as a conglomeration of untransformed beta elements. And it is only when we reach this level of functioning that structural change can take effect.

CHAPTER 12

Bion's theory of containment

RUTH RIESENBERG-MALCOLM

Bion is one of the most influential psychoanalytic figures in the second half of this century. Following Sigmund Freud and Melanie Klein, he developed the latter's theories in one of the most original ways, thus opening up vast fields of understanding of the functioning of the human mind, mental development and psychopathology. He applied his newly discovered theories to further psychoanalytic technique and the understanding of groups.

His writings may appear difficult and obscure at first reading, but they manage to inspire the reader. For the practising analyst they help to refine and expand technical expertise.

Bion was born in India in 1897. As a young boy he was sent to boarding school in England. He finished school just before the outbreak of the First World War. He soon joined the army, where he distinguished himself in the Royal Tank Corps and received the DSO. At the end of the war he went to Oxford to read History. Then, after a short period of school-teaching, he decided to study Medicine and specialize in Psychiatry.

In 1940 he again enrolled in the army, where he looked after psychiatric war casualties. Together with Rickman, Main, Foulks and others, he worked on the rehabilitation of war personnel. Bion became very interested in what he observed as the group processes that were taking place in the wards he worked in, and he began to observe and study the possible meanings of the patients' interactions, and the possibility of using this newly acquired under-standing as a therapeutic tool.

Eventually this working group of psychiatrists formed the Institute of Human Relations of the Tavistock Clinic.

Bion's work with groups allowed him to bring to being the first of his many original contributions which appeared in 1961 as the book *Experiences in Groups*. In this book he describes what he calls the 'basic assumptions', that is the processes that underlie the emotional interaction in groups. These assumptions are Fight and Flight, Dependency and Pairing. I will not go into group phenomena in this chapter, but I wish to stress that having been in analysis with Rickman (analysis he had to interrupt because of their work together during the war), Bion was aware of Melanie Klein's ideas. Later on he was to analyse his own ideas about groups from a Kleinian perspective (Bleandonu, 1994, p. 84). His work on groups was not only illuminating, but to this day remains central to the understanding of group phenomena and to work with groups.

In 1945, Bion went into analysis with Melanie Klein, whose theories he later expanded on and enriched with new ideas. Klein's insights into early mental functioning, and especially her discovery and description of the mechanism of projective identification, her theories about the depressive and paranoid-schizoid position and the movement between them, were to become central to Bion's thinking. These can be found in Klein's 'Notes on some schizoid mechanisms' (1946).

The focus of this paper will be what has become known as Bion's theory of 'containment' or 'container and contained'. I consider this to be his most important contribution to psychoanalysis because, in my view, it takes Melanie Klein's original idea of projective identification and expands it in such a way as to make it essential for the understanding of normal as well as pathological development.

I would define the theory of containment as the capacity of one individual (or object) to receive in himself projections from another individual, which he then can sense and use as communications (from him), transform them, and finally give them back (or convey back) to the subject in a modified form. Eventually, this can enable the person (an infant at first) to sense and tolerate his own feelings and develop a capacity to think.

Before expanding on this subject, I wish to illustrate my definition with a brief example from a patient I treated a long time ago. [This clinical case has been published in my book *On Bearing Unbearable States of Mind,* Malcolm (1999).]

Example: Jim

Jim, a 13-year-old boy, was sent for treatment by his school because he soiled himself. The problem had reached such a stage that the school felt unable to tolerate it or him any longer. Other than his soiling he was no 'trouble' at school, but he did not relate or speak to anyone, be it child or adult. He could use speech, and understand it and was also able to read and write. His mother, a closed-in woman with an air of discontent, said he soiled at home at night and that he had always been a withdrawn boy. She gave no further information.

Jim was thin and small for his age and wore a permanent 'angelical smile' on his face. He did not put up any resistance to coming into the room, nor did he show any sign of being aware of my presence. He just sat rigidly in front of me, and for a time he did not respond to me at all or seem to notice the world outside him; it was as if he were enveloped in his 'angelical smile'.

Some time later, and with encouragement from me, he finally took some paper and a black crayon and covered half of the sheet with messy scrawling black strokes. While this was going on (for weeks and weeks), I was puzzled, though not anxious. I felt that he was conveying something awful to me, the nature of which I knew not. At times I felt very sorry for him, but curiously not bored in spite of the repetitiveness of the situation.

I spoke to him of him feeling something black, incomprehensible, inside himself. I also spoke of his not expecting me to understand or make sense of this. For several weeks I could detect no response. I spoke little while he went on blackening the page. I attempted to verbalize my communications in different ways. Sometimes I linked it to his symptom. In spite of the apparent lack of response and the repetitiveness I did not feel disconnected from Jim.

After some time I received some oblique glances from him, and I noticed that the smile was not there.

Finally, in one session, after occupying himself for a while with his usual scribbling, and when about two-thirds of the sheet was a solid black mess, he drew two circles in the blank space left on the paper. The circles were clearly delineated, separated from each other and attached by the ream to the black mass. He did not fill them in. This made me think of the lights of a car and I said so to him. He nodded. Then I told him that my words threw some light either on the mess he seemed to be in, or that he felt he had inside him, and that he was now experiencing some slight hope that together we could understand this. It was more or less at this point that he stopped using paper and crayon and began to talk.

I have brought in this example to illustrate how something is being 'put by one person into another person'. In Jim's case a sense of utter incomprehensibility and despair, and possibly many other things as well, about which I shall not speculate here. Incomprehensibility, be it his or mine, was 'felt and sensed by me' and I allowed him to convey it to me and me to feel it, while trying to make sense of it and to describe this to him.

Containment

I have chosen the concept of 'containment' as the centre of this paper, since it is at the base of Bion's main contributions, such as the understanding of: (a) psychoses, (b) emotional development, (c) thinking and learning, and (d) psychoanalytic technique.

In speaking about containment I am referring to Bion's use of Klein's concept of projective identification (Klein, 1946, pp. 8–11; see also Chapter

9). I will use here Elizabeth Spillius' very clear description of Klein's usage of the concept of projective identification:

> She [Klein] thought of projective identification as a phantasy in which bad parts of the self were split off from the rest of the self and, together with bad excrements, were projected into the mother or her breast to control and take possession of her in such a fashion that she was felt to *become* [italics in the original] the bad self. Good parts of the self were projected too, she thought, leading to the enhancement of the ego and of good object relations, providing the process was not carried to excess. (Spillius, 1988a, Vol. 1, p. 81)

Let me now return to Bion. Bion arrived at the concept of container and contained mainly from his studies of psychotic patients, their mental functioning and, very specifically, their peculiar thinking. During the sessions, Bion saw the patients expressing something they could not understand nor 'sense' themselves. It was then left to the analyst to do something with the unassimilated 'stuff' in her own mind (as I have shown in the case of Jim) and to try to convey what was happening via interpretation in such a way that it could be felt and thought by the patient.

This furthering of Klein's ideas expanded and changed the concept of projective identification itself, giving it further texture and depth, and applied it in his psychoanalytic work. This allowed him to construct a theory of infantile mental development.

Using Klein's insights, and his development of them, Bion suggests that the baby has sensations, be those coming from outside herself or from inside, which the baby cannot cope with. He counts both pleasure and pain among such sensations. Since the baby cannot 'tolerate them' (for whatever reason) or comprehend them, she can only get rid of them, that is expel them, or rather expel that bit of her that feels them (as Klein says when describing projective identification). The baby can breathe them out, she can urinate, she can scream them out or use any kind of physical means at her disposal.

A question that could be asked is: what happens with the sensations she expels, where do they go? It is obvious that in reality they cannot 'disappear', it is equally obvious that there can be no growth, well-being or development without modification.

Where do these projected bits of experience go? They go into the mother who modifies them through an emotional function that transforms the baby's raw sensations into something that – if all goes well – the baby takes back into herself and becomes the basis for the baby's awareness of her feelings and, eventually, thoughts. At first, of course, the baby cannot do this by herself, and it has to be done by the mother through a function which Bion calls 'reverie' and describes as a function of the mother that is based on her love for her baby – and the baby's father (1962b).

Reverie is an emotional experience in which the mother does something for her baby akin to 'mental digestion' (the model used by Bion), which the baby cannot do for herself. In other words the mother becomes 'a container' for the baby's experience. What the mother does is the mental equivalent to what other species do with food before giving it to their offspring. Reverie is thus an unconscious activity of the mother.

So far I have been speaking of the mother processing the baby's experience, but what does she give back to her baby? And how does she do it?

Bion describes this process by quoting Klein and the role she ascribes to an aspect of projective identification through which the baby's fears are dealt with by being projected into the good breast. Bion (1962b, p. 90) says: 'During their sojourn in the good breast [mother] they are felt to have been modified in such a way that the object that is re-introjected has become tolerable to the infant's psyche.'

I believe that Bion's statement makes it clear that the sensation, as well as the object – that is the infant's perceptions of and what he takes from the mother – become tolerable. In my view, Bion is saying that the baby takes in (unconsciously) not only the modified version of that 'him + sensation' that has been projected into the mother, but also the object, that is 'the mother in her function'. If all goes well, this will constitute the basis for further development. I will return later to the processes that take place.

Reverie as a function is central to the baby's life, but it does not only take place in infancy, it occurs as well in later life. Moreover, it is a process that takes place – or should do so – more or less continually in psychoanalytic work.

For instance, looking back at Jim's case, what I was doing was not just tolerating his behaviour or receiving his projections, I was trying to make some sense of them, and of the feelings he elicited in me, to convey whatever sense I could to him.

Bion understood reverie as a conjoined activity of baby and mother, for the mutual benefit of both. Something akin to this process takes place in the psychoanalytic session, but it is not quite the same. If we look once again to Jim; I was responding, mostly, though not exclusively, unconsciously to my perceptions of him and myself. I tried to understand what I felt and thought, process it intellectually as well as emotionally, and somehow find a way to communicate it to Jim, in such a form that conveyed to him that it was possible to make sense out of this 'amorphous mess'. He eventually took this in and could use it himself – something he demonstrated by moving towards a more sophisticated (symbolic) way of communication: the drawing of the circles and speech.

Bion's ideas on containment show us how the environment (which for the baby is at first just the mother) works through the maternal reverie in helping or hindering the baby's development.

Containment has become a popular and popularized concept, often misused. We often hear the expression 'she or he was so containing', referring to someone's capacity to bear something or some person.

I hope that in this brief introduction to the process of transforming mental elements, I have conveyed that 'containment' is an active process, which involves two people in an emotional relationship. This needs to be emphasized and kept in mind since it is a concept that is often misunderstood.

Similarly Bion's idea of containment has often been compared to Winnicott's concept of holding, however I understand them as different processes which, in spite of sharing similar experiences in descriptive terms, are understood differently.

I shall briefly explain my understanding of the main differences between Winnicott's idea of holding and Bion's concept of containing.

Following Freud, Winnicott bases 'holding' on the concept of primary narcissism, that is, no ego existence at the onset of life. He claims that baby and mother merge and fuse, and that the process of holding includes 'especially the physical holding of infant, which is a form of loving. It is perhaps the only way in which a mother can show the infant her love' (1960, p. 49). He adds that the identification of the mother with her baby allows her to provide ordinary holding.

Bion, on the other hand, followed Klein and departed from Freud's view on primary narcissism and propounds the existence of innate drives and an innate rudimentary ego capable of rudimentary functions (responses) (see Chapters 2, 3 and 11).

To summarize: both Bion and Winnicott share descriptively a view of a close mother–infant relationship, but they differ in their interpretation of this relationship. For Winnicott it is a merger, as expressed in holding, which follows the intrauterine unity between baby and mother and from which the baby emerges into eventual individualization when she is well and ready for it. For Bion (and Klein) it is a relationship between the two in which the infant's ego's participation is active from the beginning and the mother's participation is more psychologically specific than just mere physical contact, though it is mainly perceived and expressed by it.

I will now describe in more detail how this psychological transformation takes place.

Alpha-function, alpha-elements and beta-elements

In working with psychotic patients, Bion came to the realization that they had sensations, perceptions, or mental states that they could not process in themselves. They could neither feel them within themselves nor be conscious of them. Bion recalls feeling under certain pressure to 'take those states in', that is they were projected into him and it was for him to experience them. The actual aims of those patients in projecting into him, seem to have been manifold, predominantly the patients' need to get rid of something. In patients more connected to reality, these projections represented means of reaching their object, that is the analyst in the session (or mother originally) had to experience it for the patient to be able to do something about them.

In examining his own experience and action in such situations, Bion came to realize that he was doing something with what had been deposited in him, that to sense it and to make sense of it, he had to transform it into a different category of mental element. For example, apparently incomprehensible words, grunts or strange movements of his psychotic patients became bits of possible understandable material. He called the product of this mental activity alpha-elements.

Bion calls these raw sensations, which need to be dealt with (and fail to be dealt with) by alpha-function, beta-elements. Beta-elements are only fit for expulsion, or action; they cannot become thoughts or develop in the way they are; they can only be thrown out. But, as I will explain later, when these expulsions are too massive and not dealt with by alpha-function they can result in severe pathology.

Alpha-elements are created by a special function that is called by Bion alpha-function. He keeps the concept of alpha-function as an abstraction: it is a function only aimed at creating alpha-elements. The understanding of alpha-function is based on the extension and application of Klein's ideas on projective identification.

Returning to my original point on reverie, the mother (and the analyst in the session) uses her own alpha-function to transform the infant's raw sensations and raw emotions (for instance the fear of death) into something that can eventually be assimilated by the infant or patient in her own mind and become elements for further development.

Once alpha-elements are taken in by the baby (the maternal function has been introjected as well) she can use them as building blocks for emotional and intellectual development.

At the beginning of this paper I affirmed that Bion's theory of containment was also known as 'the container' and 'the contained'. By receiving the projections of beta-elements, and working them by her own alpha-function, the mother/analyst is 'a container' for these projections, which then can be called 'the contained'. Once alpha-function has converted beta-elements into alpha-elements and the mother returns these new elements to their original 'sender', they become the contained, and the baby or patient, the container.

Example

I will now introduce a vignette from the material of the analysis of a considerably disturbed woman patient that I believe illustrates this process (this case appears in my book *On Bearing Unbearable States of Mind*). The patient was a few months into her analysis and at that time I did not know much about the nature of her disturbance. During Ms X's sessions, I began to realize that I was becoming extremely curious about whatever she said, regardless of its content. It was not the usual 'analytic' curiosity about meaning or even about the subject she might be referring to, on the contrary it did not seem to be connected to any particular thing she was talking about. For instance in a session she might be saying that Peter or Anne came into her office and I would feel curious about that. Ms X worked as secretary in a laboratory and the people she mentioned were technicians that worked there. I did not know them, nor had I heard anything remarkable about them in her associations. My curiosity felt inappropriate. I asked myself what could be more natural than going into the secretary's office for everyday necessities of work. She spoke about these everyday events in a rather faltering way, I felt confused. The patient, however, did not seem confused, on the contrary, she seemed to be following a clear line of thought. If I tried to question her she responded in an excited and histrionic way. Gradually it began to emerge with some clarity in my mind that I was *supposed* to be very curious and excited by *something* that was happening in her. Something in the situation I was supposed to be witnessing was presented as possessing fascinating qualities which were meant to act as a temptation for me and compel me to join in 'something'.

This I interpreted in a rather blind manner, since I did not know what the situation was, nor the meaning of the fascination that it was meant to excite in me, despite being well aware that this was going on.

Through the continuous interpretation of this behaviour the patient began to experience me differently and I became for her a more trustworthy analyst, able to 'contain' her problems. That is, I could feel them and think about them without being reduced to act them out and, therefore, help her to understand them herself.

What then emerged was that for most of her adult life she had had a compulsive perverse masturbatory fantasy, of a voyeuristic-exhibitionistic nature which plagued her.

I believe this example illustrates two main points in relation to this theory. In projecting 'her fantasy' into me she managed to elicit a strange curiosity in me (the voyeuristic aspect of it). In the actual fantasy the voyeurs were useless. Even without knowing what it was, by being able to sense it and then describe it to her, I allowed her to take in – that is introject – a different kind of phenomenon that appertained to alpha-function and alpha-elements, which she then could use herself in linking what I said to the fantasy and to tell me about it. She did not need to project them (at least not so much) and in her mind we could both address the problem and thus the beginning of a different way of functioning could emerge.

The second point I wish to illustrate, is the process that takes place in the transformation of projections, or beta-elements, into something thinkable that is alpha-elements.

With Ms X, I seemed very much at sea for some time. But something started imposing itself in my mind, at first dimly, and then slowly with more clarity, that this was the 'strange curiosity' I felt. This sensing centred my experience of the sessions, and permitted me to address it so as to introduce a meaning of what was going on for me as well as for my patient.

I think this centring of the emotional experience, which takes place in ordinary analytic sessions, is similar to what happens in the mother's mind during reverie when she is transforming the baby's projections into alpha-elements. For instance the crying of a very small baby is responded to by the mother in different ways according to what she senses.

Bion calls this phenomenon 'the selected fact'. In his book *Learning from Experience* he quotes Poincaré's description of the process of creation of a mathematical formulation: 'If a new result is to have any value, it must unite elements long since known, but till then scattered and seemingly foreign to each other, and suddenly introduce order where the appearance of disorder reigned' (1962a, p. 72). Further on he says: 'I have used the term "selected fact" to describe that which the psycho-analyst must experience in the process of synthesis.' He then adds: 'The selected fact is the name of an emotional experience, the emotional experience of a sense of discovery of coherence' (Bion, 1962a, p. 73).

The emotional experience I am referring to, is the emotional experience the mother has when 'sensing' her baby's projections and allowing them to come together in herself in a way such that she can transform them into alpha-elements and respond to her baby, or in the case of the analyst when a formulation emerges in his mind.

I have been describing the transformation by alpha-function into alpha-elements. The fact that raw sensations can be modified and converted into elements that can be felt and assimilated suggests that they can cohere and develop into what becomes a structure. Bion calls this structure 'contact barrier'.

A contact barrier is a combination of alpha-elements that eventually can become permanent albeit elastic and can manifest itself, for instance, in a kind of narrative, such as that of a dream.

The development of a contact barrier is at the base of the differentiation between an 'unconscious' and a 'conscious'. It keeps them separate from one another, but it also allows certain permeability between them, permitting a selected passage of elements from one to the other. 'The term "contact-barrier" emphasizes the contact between conscious and unconscious' (Bion, 1962b, p. 17). An everyday example of this is that when we are reading a book we can, as it were, keep out of our mind the fact that we have to telephone someone. Both can easily be brought in different order into mind, when necessary. Of course it is different when we speak of different kinds of unconscious processes which require a special mental work to be brought into the realm of consciousness, as for instance the meaning of a dream or in Ms X's case, the meaning of her projections into her analyst and their relationship to basic conflicts in her life. In an analysis we are continuously examining both the conscious content of the patient's expressions, as well as trying to elucidate their possible unconscious signification.

As I said before, the beta-elements do not develop, and therefore cannot cohere. But they can agglutinate, in a way that sometimes masquerades as a coherence that does not exist. Bion calls this a beta-screen.

Beta-screen does not allow the separation between a 'conscious' and an 'unconscious'. Bion suggests that there is a kind of division, but with an indiscriminate passage of elements from one area to the other. Clinically, the beta-screen presents itself to observation as akin to a confusional or psychotic state, for example, through an outpouring of disjointed phrases and images which are related more to the patient's need to produce an emotional involvement in the analyst than a psychoanalytic interpretation.

Bion says: 'Beta screen ... has a quality enabling it to evoke the kind of response the patient desires, or, alternatively, a response from the analyst which is heavily charged with counter-transference' (Bion, 1962a, p. 23).

I have quoted this statement mainly to emphasize that beta-elements are only prone to be projected, and therefore, can evoke in their receptor (the analyst in the session) those emotions, feelings or sensations that have been ejected. Bion's second statement is more complicated, since it refers mainly to Bion's use of the word 'countertransference', with which he seems to imply a neurotic (personal response) from the analyst.

I understand Bion's last remark in two ways. On the one hand that the analyst has been provoked and has not been able to process his own reactions. On the other, what he describes as the provocation of a desired response of the analyst, which in modern psychoanalytic technique has become known as 'the use of the countertransference'. In other words, the use of the understanding of the patient's projections and the reactions they provoke as means of the patients' communications. We could see this in Ms X's 'making me feel curious'. It is interesting to note that such an understanding of countertransference has occurred and has produced such a vast development in psychoanalytic technique thanks to Bion's theories.

However, the way we currently use the word countertransference is different from the meaning that Bion gives to it in the cited paragraph. It is impossible to gauge if he would have agreed with the extension of the use of the word of countertransference, an extension due to his contributions.

Revision of theories derived from containment

As I said at the beginning of this chapter, I have focused on Bion's theory of containment because it is at the centre of the most important developments brought by Bion to psychoanalytic understanding. I will now refer briefly to three theories that developed from containment: 'theory of thinking', the development of 'knowledge' (as derived from the previous one), and a few of his contributions to the understanding of psychoses.

Before developing these aspects I wish to remind the reader that Bion follows Freud and Klein in his adherence to the existence of innate life and death drives. He uses these concepts (as they both did) in his theoretical refinements, and in explaining clinical phenomena, especially the influence of destructiveness in the origins of psychoses as well as the type of mental phenomena involved in psychotic development.

Bion departs from Freud in his ideas about primary narcissism (as I mentioned earlier) and believes in the existence of a rudimentary ego (as did Klein) and that the individual was born with a preconception of a satisfying object, that is the breast (see Chapter 8).

Bion believed that the capacity for development depends greatly on the subject's capacity to tolerate frustration, which in turn depends on the innate, instinctive destructive forces.

Theory of thinking

Bion suggests that thinking and thoughts, though not independent from one another, develop differently and suggests that thoughts develop independently of, and prior to, thinking. Thinking he considered to be an apparatus that the individual needed to develop so as to be able to deal with thoughts.

Bion describes thought as evolving through a developmental process, that begins with what he calls preconceptions which then evolve into conceptions and eventually concepts. This is an emotional process.

He describes preconceptions as states of expectation, for instance a baby feeling hungry and expecting to be fed by the breast; this seems to be basically an instinctive psycho-physiological state. When these expectations are not met by gratification (being fed), and if frustration is not too great they can develop into conceptions. Conception is a primitive thought that results from a preconception (expectation) meeting a 'negative realization', that is the absence of the object that satisfies, added to a tolerance of this absence, without the situation turning into a catastrophe. Concepts are repeated conceptions; they can become fixed and be named.

As I said before, the infant is born with a preconception of an object that will satisfy her needs: the breast. When the breast satisfies her, no further development of that specific experience takes place, insofar as the baby is satisfied and contented. Expressed in a slightly different way the discomforted and/or hungry baby feels something bad and expels it, a beta-element is got rid into the mother who can sense it and give her baby what she understands the baby to need, she can for instance put her nipple in the infant's mouth. Thus, when a preconception meets a gratification it can be considered the end of that story.

The situation is quite different if the preconception meets with frustration. To a certain extent the outcome will depend on the infant's capacity to tolerate frustration (which has already permitted the introjection of good experiences with the mother).

To start with the negative aspect of this, when the tolerance of frustration is minimal or non-existent, the capacity for satisfaction is also impeded, since anything short of perfection will not do, and this added dissatisfaction increases the frustration, which results in continuous and massive use of projection, and re-introjection of bad unmodified beta-elements, which are felt not just to be bad, but 'even worse than bad'. Expectation, hostility and frustration grow and the introjection is of a kind of horrible stuff which installs itself in the baby's mind as a bad, negating damaging object.

Turning now to those infants with the capacity to tolerate frustration, the preconception that meets with frustration can become a conception, that is, a thought.

In the instance of the intolerance of frustration, the baby's main aim would appear to be to evade frustration. The main aim of a 'tolerant-of-frustration baby', on the other hand, would be to modify it –to think it– which in turn will increase his capacity to tolerate frustration.

To summarize: a thought derives from a bad object, felt to be bad because it is not there and therefore does not gratify the infant's need of the moment, albeit that it can be tolerated by the baby. I believe that we can assume the pre-existence of innate capacities and sufficient previous gratification by a good object that permit the infant to tolerate the situation, and eventually allow him to develop thought. For Bion, a thought that becomes fixed and can be named is a 'concept'. It could be said that by then it is firmer and better established.

Turning now to the apparatus for thinking thoughts, this presents a different and more complex situation. Bion says that this apparatus has to be formed so as to deal with thoughts, but in my reading of him I do not get a clear view of how this takes place. I will return to this soon.

In his paper 'A theory of thinking', Bion says: 'just as sense-data have to be modified and worked on by alpha-function to make them available for dream thoughts etc., so the thoughts have to be worked on to make them available for translation into action. Translation into action involves publication, communication and commonsense' (1962b, pp. 117–18).

As can be seen, Bion's idea of an apparatus for thinking follows Freud in his postulations about thought modifying simple discharges and permitting a different kind of action, according to the reality principle (Freud, 1911a).

Bion describes with great vividness the origins of the transformation of 'simple discharges', that is, projection of raw sensation or beta-elements, first by maternal reverie into alpha-elements, to evolve into what becomes a concept. From his writings one can deduce that the apparatus for thinking probably evolves from these early emotional experiences, and out of necessity, but I do not find it clear how this happens. If one is to follow his idea of an apparatus for thinking as separate from thoughts, I would have thought that it probably originates in the introjection of the maternal function as such.

It is my belief that the baby, in taking in the maternal transformation of her projections of raw sensations as transformed into alpha-elements, takes with it some of the maternal attitude and capacity to transform, that is introjects the function as well as the content. In this sense it would be the summation of these introjections that probably would permit the formation of a specific apparatus to deal with thoughts.

We can see from this description that 'intellectual activities', that is the formation of thoughts and the constitution of an apparatus for thinking, originate in emotional experiences, between the infant and its primary object and evolve from there.

Theory of knowledge: knowledge (K) and anti knowledge (minus-K)

As I suggested earlier, learning, and therefore knowledge, derives from the developments described above, which in turn are based on emotional relationships.

During most of his working life Bion was interested in facilitating notation. He felt that resorting to a few basic concepts, from which symbols could be abstracted that represent these complex relationships, facilitates the task of an analyst.

He chose three main and central relationships between the infant and his primary objects, or the patient to his analyst in the sessions. These were Love, Hate and Knowledge, which he represented with the letters L, H and K. He emphasized that the three of them constitute an active process as opposed to static statements.

Leaving aside L and H, Bion describes K (or knowledge) as a process, a continuous movement of 'coming to know'.

If we look back to what I have been saying previously about alpha-function and alpha-elements, in the same way that they continuously change, knowledge, or K, also constitutes a similar continuous process of movement and change.

This tendency to come to know (K), or what Klein refers to as the epistemophilic instinct, probably also corresponds to innate tendencies, as can be deduced from the capacities of the infant or individual to tolerate the 'frustration' of not knowing and moving towards the exploration that will permit the coming to know.

In an ordinary infant or person this activity is not only continuous but also implies growth of the personality. Early omnipotence is replaced by knowledge and the person does not have to rely on it, she can learn.

Thus, K would be based both on the mother's capacity for reverie as well as the infant's capacity to tolerate frustration.

There is however a less positive scenario which I mentioned earlier when dealing with preconceptions. I am referring to the situation in which either the mother cannot transform the baby's projections or these are of such a nature and the infant's destructive forces are so negative that instead of a positive evolution what takes place is the establishment of a destructive denuding object in the infant.

In such a situation all the positive achievements of growth (and mutual growth of object and subject) are impeded and appear to be reversed. Instead of feeling relieved by the mother's ministrations, and her capacity for reverie, which eventually could be assimilated by him, the infant experiences the maternal action as destructive of his own capacities, and suffused with hatred. When the mother removes the infant's anxieties, the infant feels her as depriving him, not giving to him. Projective identification increases, but not in a communicative way, on the contrary it is aimed at destroying communication, it appears to act as missiles, attacking whichever capacity should there be available for the production of alpha-activity.

Since projection and introjection are basic components of the infants, and they take place either simultaneously or in succession, introjections that occur are of hostile elements. Thus the individual installs inside himself an object he feels destroys him, denuding him of goodness and exposing him to moral criticism. Omnipotence and omniscience replace learning and knowledge. 'Morality' – that is to condemn everything – takes the place of 'Truth'.

Psychoses

Bion's contributions to the understanding and treatment of psychoses are vast and go beyond the scope of this chapter; nevertheless I do not wish to end it without mentioning briefly two aspects that relate directly with what has been said so far about Bion's theory of containment.

I concluded my last chapter point talking about minus-K which ushers the introduction of psychotic phenomena. This, because of the predominance of minus-K, is psychotic in nature, and the internal world of such individuals feels distorted, hostile and destructive to them.

According to Bion, psychosis (and by this he refers mainly to schizo-phrenia) originates in an excessive endowment of destructive forces, which cannot be mitigated even by the most responsive of mothers (and who can be so responsive in such situations?). Maternal lack of capacity to accept and process the baby's projections, indeed contributes to create pathology, furthering the instalment in the child of a rejecting (rejecting of projective identification) object. But Bion insists that this alone cannot create psychosis.

The infant so negatively endowed feels this endowment as hatred to all that which brings awareness (that is anything that can link her to reality), and the attacks are mainly directed to that aspect of the self that could be(come) aware of connections, both inside himself and others, and towards the object that prompts this awareness. In other words, what is being attacked and destroyed are mainly the functions of the ego. It is the ego that is being destroyed.

The attack on the ego is carried through by the minute fragmentation of the ego and by projecting these fragments violently into the object. The object might then be felt to engulf and/or be engulfed by these expelled minute bits of the self that contain beta-elements plus ego and superego (internal object) fragments (see Chapter 9).

Bion calls these particles 'bizarre objects', and as can be seen they are based on beta-elements, but are different to them insofar as beta-elements are exclusively raw sensations, while these projected bits contain also bits of ego and superego.

When writing of containment and the projective identification implicit in it, I have mainly (but not exclusively) referred to a certain capacity of the individual to elicit feelings and responses, and in this respect I have spoken of a realistic projective identification (see for instance the curiosity in the Ms X case). But in the case of a psychotic patient, the violence and hatred of connections is so intense that the projections often involve inanimate objects, which are then felt to be and act as that which was projected into them. Bion often uses the example of sight projected into a gramophone which then is felt to watch the patient.

The main and earlier mental connection between baby and mother (and patient and analyst in the sessions) is projective identification, that is the link formed by a 'realistic' projective identification: the baby has projected raw sensations, the mother has transformed them into alpha-elements, and the baby has taken them back in himself. It is this link that becomes the main target of the psychotic infant's attacks, and Bion sustains that even more effective than the attack on the links would be to prevent those links from being formed (Bion, 1959).

These attacks, as I have already said, fragment the ego and the patient is confronted with the task of restoring his own ego, prior to any kind of reparation to the object.

To conclude: for Bion projective identification is the central and most primary link between infant and mother, and the capacities of each one – mother and baby – to use it, transform and assimilate it forms the core for both normal as well as pathological development. In other words, with his theory of containment, Bion brought new lights into Melanie Klein's concept of projective identification and allowed for further understanding of the human mind, both normal as well as pathological.

CHAPTER 13

Transference

BETTY JOSEPH

By 1905 in his paper 'Fragment of an analysis of a case of hysteria' Freud had formulated his ideas on transference – ideas which are still fundamental to our understanding of the term and to our psychoanalytic technique today. He asks:

> What are transferences? They are new editions or facsimiles of the impulses and phantasies which are aroused and made conscious during the progress of the analysis ... they replace some earlier person by the person of the physician ... a whole series of psychological experiences are revived, not as belonging to the past, but as applying to the person of the physician at the present moment.

Freud sees that transference 'is an inevitable necessity' and that it is 'the one thing the presence of which has to be detected almost without assistance and with only the slightest clues to go upon'. Later analysts, particularly Melanie Klein, then worked on such issues as what is meant by these 'impulses and phantasies', 'series of psychological experiences', and how they get built up, how they get 'replaced' on to the person of the physician, the analyst, and how they may be 'detected'. Melanie Klein describes (1952b) 'in unravelling the details of the transference it is essential to think in terms of *total situations* transferred from the past into the present, as well as of emotions, defences and object relationships'.

How then do we see transference today? It becomes clear that we don't just mean that the patient treats the analyst as if he were the patient's real mother or father, but that his/her picture of the parent has been built up and internalized since infancy and that it is this picture or rather aspects of it, and these internal objects that attach themselves to the analyst in treatment (and indeed to other objects in the external world). The internal objects are not of course simply replicas of the real parents (if it were possible to visualize such

181

things as 'real parents'). These internal objects (see Chapter 8) are built up partly from the way the child was treated from the very early weeks onward – whether he was treated, for example with love and concern or harshly and coldly, how he was actually handled, fed, played with or neglected etc. But the actual handling, which is so important, is not the whole story. Something comes from the infant or child's own make up - how he responds to the handling he receives. Some infants and young children from very early on appear to respond to any disturbance or frustration with great anxiety, others seem to tolerate strain and difficulties much more easily, some will explode with rage very quickly, others are more patient, others will appear just to give in and withdraw. The picture the infant constructs of his objects from the beginning will be coloured therefore not only by what actually happens to him but by the nature of his own individual responses to his world.

We are describing here the mechanisms that not only construct the individual's inner world but continue to operate throughout life and which we can observe in operation in the relationship with the analyst – mechanisms of projection and introjection. The infant, child, the future adult and patient projects his own feelings, impulses and phantasies into his objects and then feels about them accordingly; he takes into himself, introjects, objects that are constantly being imbued with his own feelings (see Chapter 9). We observe this happening when, for example, the analyst gives an interpretation to the patient, the latter may well not hear it in the way it was intended – but as infused by his infantile experiences. We may believe we are giving an interpretation in a dispassionate way, intended to increase understanding, but the patient may hear it as a criticism or attack and therefore respond with anxiety or anger. This in itself will lead him to expect the analyst to feel hostile to him and a vicious circle will be set up, started by his false perception.

James Strachey in 1934 wrote 'The nature of the therapeutic action of psychoanalysis' basing his ideas on Klein's description of the role of projection and introjection in the analytic situation. He described how such vicious circles get established – the patient projecting his impulses and aspects of his internal world into the analyst and then reacting to the latter as if these elements were actually part of the analyst. He discussed how the analysing of such movements from moment to moment makes psychic change possible.

Freud (1905a) discussed how transferences 'replace some earlier person by the person of the physician'. We could now describe this process of 'replacing' as being an aspect of projective identification - as Melanie Klein termed it. Parts of the self and of internal objects are projected in the patient's phantasy into an object, who then becomes identified with what is projected. If we go further and enquire what is it that is being projected - we can observe that sometimes it is more a part of the ego, for example it may be the patient's capacity to think that is projected into the analyst, and the patient becomes passive and pseudo-stupid; or it may be the sense of guilt which is felt as unbearably persecuting by the patient who then tries unconsciously to rid himself of it by making the analyst feel at fault and guilty; it may be a more total situation of complex relationships where the patient will attempt to manipulate the analyst into enacting a role belonging essentially to the past but now very much part of his internal world and his unconscious expectation of his external world. Strachey puts this very neatly when in his 1934 paper he describes that the transference process gives us, the analyst:

> our great opportunity. Instead of having to deal as best we may, with conflicts of the remote past, which are concerned with dead circumstances and mummified personalities, and whose outcome is already determined, we find ourselves involved in an actual and immediate situation, in which we and the patient are the principal characters ...

Before going on to discuss some of the implications I want to bring a brief example of the kind of situation I have in mind. The patient P was a very young newly qualified and somewhat arrogant architect, who had significant difficulties in his relationships. Both parents were living, his father was seen as a very critical man who denigrated and was contemptuous towards the mother yet was clearly devoted to her. My patient and his two younger brothers joined in the denigration of the mother and she tended to submit and collude with this attitude in a quietly masochistic way. In the session I am quoting I had made a rather straightforward interpretation linking something that P had said with some understanding established in the previous session which had to do with his contemptuous attitude. My patient flared up saying something to the effect that his quarrel was not with what I said but as he put it 'how you say it'. He then just quietly moved on to describe his feelings about a Prof. X who had chaired an architectural meeting the day before; P said how he liked this man despite what other people said about him; he respected the way he could let ideas grow and develop in the meeting and yet be firm. The Professor twice told S (a lecturer in the college to which he is attached and who appears to be ageing in mind and body) to shut up when she seemed to be talking about issues which were irrelevant to the point under discussion. But afterwards he very nicely took her by the arm and helped her down the stairs to the taxi waiting for her in the street.

The way my patient describes this gives us a picture of what was going on in the session, of the transference. As the patient talks we listen both to the description of his life and activities but also to the particular content chosen. Experience points to the fact that what is selected elucidates something of the relationship to the analyst - that the material is unconsciously selected from all the other things the patient could have talked about because of its relevance to what is going on in the immediate situation. Thus my patient first tells me very brusquely to shut up when he says 'my quarrel is with how you say it'. But he then quickly becomes quiet, changes the subject, revises his picture of me, reassuring me, and thus helps me down the stairs. This I associated with the kind of contempt that we had been seeing on the previous day – how I had become the troublesome and ageing S with my irrelevant remarks and I linked it with the way he used to ally himself with his father and brothers against his mother, while remaining apparently benign but superior.

P apparently took no notice of my interpretation but went on to describe how he had received a letter from his mother enclosing an article from a newspaper on a current architectural issue, which was very much in the news at that moment, in the papers, on the radio etc. It seemed therefore somewhat unnecessary for his mother to have sent it, but my patient expressed great appreciation. I suggested that his appreciation had hidden behind it criticism and contempt towards his mother for thinking that it would be worthwhile sending it to him. Further I suggested that one of his conditions for appreciating and ostensibly looking up to me, his analyst, was that he could at the same time secretly look down on me and the interpretations that I had just sent/given. He could then, as with his mother, feel me to be weak and rather stupid.

In this material we can see something of the complexity and richness of what P brings into the relationship with me, how he and I become in his mind 'involved in an immediate and actual situation' in which we are 'the principal character'. When I make my first interpretation, which the patient hears as wrongly said, I am treated harshly and with contempt. But then P immediately becomes kind, shifts, tells of the meeting and the situation is described in which he is the firm Prof. X and I am the ageing S with whom he has abandoned his harsh tone and taken gently by the arm.

The interpretation seems to me significant but P disregards it and this similar scenario is simultaneously described and enacted. I have given an interpretation but though as with the newspaper article appreciation is indicated, it is treated as unnecessary. When P was angry because of what he felt to be the tone of my voice, naturally one needs to consider whether there was in the way I spoke something actually critical, or how much was this a projection of his own hypercritical self. P's fear of his own harshness and cruelty is very important as was indicated in his quick flight from open criticism of me to a benign story about the meeting. P's treating me as a weak or stupid person might be considered as primarily a projection of an internal weak figure, but in fact we can observe how P constructs me into being this kind of figure. If I do not notice that his appreciation of his mother's sending the article must be false (which later he agreed with) then I would be an easily flattered weak person, if I do I can readily be experienced as being hard.

This brief vignette highlights a number of issues – for example how does the analyst find the elements being enacted, bearing in mind Freud's statement quoted earlier when he said about transference that it is 'the one thing the presence of which has to be detected almost without assistance and with only the slightest clues to go upon'. This I touched upon at the beginning of the material from P. Melanie Klein in her 1952b paper took this issue a step further when she wrote:

> For many years ... transference was understood in terms of direct references to the analyst in the patient's material. My conception of transference as rooted in the earliest stages of development and in deep layers of the unconscious is much wider and entails a technique by which from the whole material presented the *unconscious elements* of the transference are deduced. For instance, reports of patients about their everyday life, relations and activities not only give insight into the functioning of the ego, but also reveal – if we expose their unconscious content – the defences against the anxieties stirred up in the transference situation.

In his description of the meeting P demonstrates certain important anxieties and the nature of his defences against them. First how any interpretation that is felt to disturb his own picture of himself stirs anger, this makes him anxious and has to be smoothed down in a placatory way – as we see in his anger with me being evaded by his turning to the story of the meeting, and the criticism of the ageing S being quickly followed by the flattery and kindness of Prof. X. P's deep fear of the intensity or cruelty of his aggression, drives him to a defensive manoeuvre of placating and flattering his object. His narcissism is constantly threatened by the analytic situation where the analyst has the professional/superior role and this leads to a defensive attempt to assert himself against interpretations or disregard them. His anxiety about feeling small or dependent plays into his need to assert his superiority and thus we get a series of interlocking vicious circles. The connection between the way of operating that we see in this vignette and his history of the men in his family ganging up against and humiliating the mother was clear, but behind this I think is the picture of a child whose unconscious rivalry with and envy of a creative parent is starting more clearly to emerge.

It is not only through direct references to figures of the past, or as I have just indicated, reports about the patient's everyday life, that the analyst gains clues about the nature of the transference, but in addition we learn from what we feel is going on, is being enacted, in the session and this can often largely be gauged from the analyst's monitoring, not only what the patient is saying and how he is saying it, but also what is being stirred up in the analyst's own feelings – what we would nowadays broadly call his counter-transference. Freud in his writings rarely used the word 'countertransfer-ence' and where he did he largely saw it as a negative force, something in the analyst's relationship with his patient that arose from an insufficiently analysed, more disturbed part of his personality. Freud writes in one of his papers on technique (1915c) 'Observations on transference love', 'In my opinion therefore we ought not to give up the neutrality to the patient which we have acquired through keeping the countertransference in check.' But by the 1950s there was much interest in the more positive under-standing and use of countertransference, significant contributions being made for example by Heimann in her paper of 1950 'On countertransfer-ence', and Racker (1968). Klein herself scarcely alludes directly to counter-transference but her work on projective identification has of course played a fundamental part in the understanding of countertransference over the last three or four decades.

As I have discussed, our patients bring into the relationship with the analyst their internal world, their archaic ways of relating – but what effect does this have on the analyst, can he just remain 'neutral'? What responses does he make? This is the stuff of countertransference. The majority of analysts nowadays, I believe, would agree that the task of the analyst is not just to 'check' in the sense of hold back, ward off, the countertransference but to keep a check on it – to monitor what is aroused in him- or herself and locate where it comes from. He needs to sort out whether what is aroused comes mainly from something in his own personality – anxieties, defences that have been touched off by something in the session; whether it arises mainly from the patient and what he is trying, consciously or unconsciously to arouse in the analyst and manipulate the analyst into enacting. The pull towards enactment is probably constant, patient and analyst subtly affecting each other all the time – it may be very subtle, the analyst for example may only realize that he felt critical and was a bit condemning in his attitude when he hears his voice becoming slightly sarcastic, or that he has become too identified with his patient when he realizes that his voice or words seem particularly 'understanding'.

The patient's material may push the analyst into becoming actually defen-sive, the analyst allowing himself to be manipulated into a position that is more comfortable both for himself and his patient, avoiding confronting what is currently going on. This kind of pressure can be seen in the brief description of the young architect P. It would be very much more comfort-able for the analyst – and patient – for the analyst not to pick up and interpret, say, the quick shift from anger and criticism to the placatory story about the meeting, to leave it and remain a benign object. We all want to be liked and having to stand up to anxiety, possible hostility, regret, threatens our defences. Sometimes of course the risk of enactment is of the opposite kind – when the patient tries consciously or unconsciously to manipulate the analyst into losing his temper or joining into a kind of argumentative quasi-interpretative struggle, or overt sado-masochistic behaviour, a type of pressure that was very important at times with P. Our patients can most subtly, unconsciously discover the analyst's defences, weak spots and play into them.

These various considerations take us into the heart of what Bion described as containment – the importance of the analyst being able to tolerate, contain, whatever the patient brings into the relationship with him, so that the analyst is in a state of mind in which he can become aware of what the patient is projecting into him, without unduly reacting to it (see Chapter 12). 'Unduly' because as I have indicated, it may be almost impossible for the analyst to register such projections until he has noticed himself responding to them, however slightly. As I have described, it is essential that the analyst checks on his feelings and ideas to help him to distinguish what has not been projected by the patient but has arisen from his own personality, impulses or defences. Yet there is an additional point that needs to be made: while an understanding of countertransference is of very great importance, the attention of the analyst must of necessity be primarily on the patient and what is going on in him; any preoccupation by the analyst with his own feelings or phantasies suggests that contact with and understanding of the patient is getting lost.

Earlier in this chapter I suggested that if one thought of behaviour that the patient brought into the relationship with the analyst as just a replica of his 'actual' past I could not see how real psychic change could be achieved. One might get changes in behaviour or ways of responding but inner, psychic change requires more than this. It involves a shifting in emotions and impulses, a change in the relationship between different aspects of the self – we might describe this as between the ego and the superego – or to take this further – a change in the relationship between the patient's internal objects and parts of the self. Change and movement can be observed by the analyst as happening in the session, interpretations will then help the patient to observe himself and thus make contact with such shifts and become aware of fragments of emotional experience deriving from unconscious sources that would ordinarily not be available to him. As the analyst tracks these shifts in the patient, or the pressures put on the analyst to join in, argue etc. there will be movement – gratitude for understanding may emerge and the analyst be felt as understanding and benign, and momentarily be internalized as such; or as we saw with the architect P understanding may be bypassed, suggesting that as it comes from the analyst it disturbs the patient and stirs up his rivalry.

So it has to be disregarded and the analyst kept redundant and stupid. Then a different kind of object is introjected, weak and hostile. As these minute shifts are not only observed but experienced by the patient, we can get what Strachey described as a 'breach in the vicious circle'. It is these vicious circles that manifest themselves as constant repetitions of unsatisfactory patterns of behaviour and mood.

There is only one way in which we can really begin to breach these vicious circles, that is through interpretations. The patterns of behaviour may appear to alter without any interpretations being given by the analyst – as when P moved away quickly from his quietly attacking behaviour to talk of other things. But this kind of shift leads to no change within the personality, only to defensive flight from his impulses and a splitting in his picture of the object, the analyst who then, for example, becomes benign, possibly ideal-ized, or weak but harmless. If we can follow and put into words the kind of movement in the relationship between patient and analyst as I have been describing, both patient and analyst can observe what is going on – the shifts and change in impulses, emotions and defences. It is this that helps us to understand how the transference is constructed because it is re-happening in the consulting room. I suspect that any techniques that do not depend on interpretation necessarily mean that the analyst or therapist is trying, consciously or not, to 'influence' the patient by projecting his own values, ambitions, judgments etc. into the patient. And this, so far as is humanly possible, psychoanalysis aims to avoid.

To illustrate this I shall bring brief material from an adolescent patient, Jenny, aged 16 – she was stuck in her development and had no interests in life apart from watching films and video. Her mother seemed a devoted but over-anxious and intrusive person, her father kindly but weak. Jenny described awful fights with her parents but with me appeared pleasant and agreeable – however it soon became clear that she would apparently accept anything I said, seemingly agree with it but nothing much moved in the analysis. The material I want to bring comes from a period when there had been some shift in this and she was studying better and had actually obtained a place at a college just outside London. I managed to rearrange her times to fit in with the college schedule; she first agreed to them but within a few days she decided that she only wanted to come three days a week instead of four and not on Tuesdays at 5.00 p.m.

On the following session, a Monday, Jenny said she had been worrying all over the weekend about this question of the Tuesday sessions; she seriously did not want to come at 5.00 p.m. – she resented it and wanted me to go along with her point of view. I agreed that it made her feel guilty not to come and she wanted me to remove the sense of guilt. She went on to describe how on the previous day she and her family had decided to go to the cinema;

she had wanted to see a particular film, but her sister had wanted a different one; finally they all went to the latter, and it wasn't so bad. I explained that she wanted me to be like a little sister who doesn't disagree with her. I should see things, the films, the whole issue of the times, in the same way as she does, so that there would be no difference between us and no conflict. With difficulty Jenny managed to explain more about why she so much did not want to come on the Tuesdays. She didn't want to cling to four times a week: it was a bit suffocating; she was frightened that it would make her completely dependent, and she always felt she had to talk things over with me and get my approval before doing anything.

Here one can see a clear picture that this girl has of me – not as of someone trying to help her to find her own mind and her own interests – but as someone invasive and suffocating. She described how she feels that she gets what she calls 'explanations' from me as to what I would like, but actually she continues to do what she wants and there is no change. The analyst, in other words, may believe she is helping the patient to think and talk things over but my patient hears me as forcing my ideas on to her and actually taking over her mind. Then the only thing she can do is either to agree and apparently let herself be taken over but secretly continue to do what she wants, or run away, avoid Tuesday sessions, those are the alternatives. Talking to gain understanding from her point of view is simply not on.

So on the following day, the Tuesday, Jenny as she had planned did not come. On the Wednesday she said she was feeling guilty and annoyed by what she called 'our difference of opinion' over the issue of the Tuesday session. She said she was not going to change her mind but she had not realized how upset she would get. Ordinarily she added she does not listen to what people say and she reminded me that when I had first suggested the Tuesday 5.00 p.m. session, she had said OK, but this is what she had done all her life – just agreeing. But she added it doesn't mean a thing, I feel suffocated but I put up with it.

If we look at the nature of the transference here we can see how this patient cannot really listen or take anything in from her object, she acts agreeably enough but the object cannot really influence her in any helpful way – and as she says 'it doesn't mean a thing'. The deep anxiety seems to be that if she lets the object, now myself, in at all she will be taken over and suffocated. In a later session Jenny made clear that she believes that people are always taken in by her agreeableness.

There is here a clear example of the kind of pull towards enactment on the analyst's part that I discussed earlier. Jenny was exerting considerable pressure on me to enact the role of a weak person who would 'give in' for the sake of peace or out of apparent kindness, it would have been easier in one sense, both for patient and analyst. An alternative role would have been to respond by pushing guilt into the patient who might then have felt pressurized into coming on the Tuesdays. Or one might have been manipulated into getting frustrated and reacting with anger, and thus trying to force her to change her mind. In a way I think Jenny might have found this easier, she would have had a 'reason' to rebel and fight – any of these enactments on the analyst's part would have enabled the patient to evade the main issue of facing and understanding her underlying anxieties and her need to find her own mind.

Thus Jenny's struggle about the Tuesdays *could be* seen as a normal adolescent's struggle for independence and therefore just accepted as such. But this, as I have indicated, would not be the psychic truth. Her conflict was one aspect of her deep anxieties about the nature of her mother/analyst's over-protectiveness/invasiveness and this had first to be recognized and its unconscious elements unravelled. To give in to the notion of healthy independence would be much easier for the analyst and on one level for the patient but it would mean abandoning one's role as her analyst and seriously letting her down. It might look like kindness but would in fact be a great unkindness.

I have so far spoken about transference in adults or near adults, but I want now briefly to discuss how we see transference in the very young child. This takes us into an area about which there has been considerable controversy especially in the 1920s and '30s. Anna Freud believed that the very young child did not make a transference to the analyst because of his/her very close relationship with the actual parents – these views were later to some extent modified. Melanie Klein thought that the child began to build up an inner world of objects from the beginning of life and that aspects of this would be projected into the analyst whatever the age of the patient (see Chapter 1). It meant that Klein felt that even very young children could be treated by analytic methods.

I shall bring material from the second week of the analysis of a boy G who was then just three years old. He came to treatment because of very severe anxieties in almost all areas of his life, especially at that period focusing round defecation and he was very controlling and uncontrollable. He was however beginning to be able to let his mother bring him into the playroom and then leave him there with me while she waited for him in the waiting room upstairs. On the Thursday of the second week he came with his mother to the playroom but when she left he started to cry and shout for her. This time I had the impression that the crying was more to do with his need to force his object to give in to him than about real anxiety about losing her. So I prevented him from leaving the room and talked to him about his need to control me. He threw himself on the floor, yelled and kicked, but it was as if some part of him wanted to settle and use the playroom and material while another part forced him to go on with the wild behaviour. The violence I suggested made him more anxious as if I and the room became bad and frightening. He seemed to listen but went back to the yelling and thrashing around on the floor. The following day he came to the playroom willingly with a roll of Smarties and some bubble gum. He ate the Smarties and chewed a piece of gum. I explained that he had felt very angry with me yesterday, but today felt different and he brought some sweetness with him. He removed the gum from his mouth and gently put it in my hand. He got up and went to one of the small chairs that stand by the low playroom table and rocked it. As the seat was under the table naturally it did not fall, he rocked at it again and it remained steady, he repeated this with the other chairs. I interpreted that he was relieved that I did not give in to him yesterday but remained firm and steady like the chairs and did not let him overwhelm me. G then went on to other activities and when the session ended he left in a friendly way saying goodbye.

I think that here G demonstrates something of his internal world and his own anxieties – his determination to force his object to give in, his violence when he does not get his way and how the violence increases his anxiety so that both analyst and playroom become persecuting, and then he needs to get away, escape. By the second session we see more clearly his fear that he can overwhelm his objects (as indeed I believe he had reason to fear with his parents who were often in despair) but he also shows some capacity for affection and sweetness and some trust in his object that she can take what comes out of him (the gum and all it may represent) and can contain, remain steady and stand up to him. I am suggesting therefore that this young child brings into the new relationship with the analyst old patterns of relationships, now already part of his internal world, and colouring his expectations of his new objects. He anticipates that the analyst will be forced to collapse and will be like a weak parent. But this is not his only version of an internal figure; he seems able to find, I believe re-find, in the analyst a different and firmer object which at that moment he clearly values.

Once Freud had discovered the existence and significance of transference, psychoanalytic technique had been influenced for ever. With Klein's contribution to the understanding of the formation of the inner world and how this becomes projected, transferred into the analytic relationship, psychoanalysis took a major step forward.

It made the previously powerful dependence on the patient's history avoidable. What our patients tell us about their history is always of interest and significance. But the issue becomes whether we listen to the patient's account of his past to explain his pathology, or whether we listen to it as we listen to all his other communications – as indicating something going on in the present, asking ourselves why did it come up now? is it because it illuminates a new piece of understanding? is it a flight from some immediate anxiety in the current relationship? or many other things. It is not of course that the analyst is not concerned about the patient's external life and happenings, his other relationships, but if we can start from the current situation, the patient's feelings and ways of relating in the session, then it becomes possible to understand how this may be reflected in the outside world and in his external relationships, and the interpretations can fan out accordingly, or the patient himself may begin to make these connections, verbally or just as shifts in feelings towards and about people.

I have tried in this chapter to discuss the meaning of transference and how it derives not just from the patient's past but from his inner world. This inner world is built up from the beginning of life, from his actual experiences interwoven with his own impulses and phantasies. What is transferred colours the relationship between patient and analyst constantly exerting pressure, subtle or gross, on the analyst to enact some role. It is the detailed understanding of this relationship - transference/countertransference - that emerges as central to psychoanalytic technique.

References

Abraham K (1911) Notes on the psycho-analytical investigation and treatment of manic-depressive insanity and allied conditions. In E Jones (ed.) Selected Papers of Karl Abraham. London: Hogarth Press, 1942, 137-56.

Abraham K (1919) A particular form of neurotic resistance against the psycho-analytic method. In E Jones (ed.) Selected Papers on Psycho-Analysis. London: Maresfield Reprints (1979), 303-17.

Abraham K (1920) Manifestations of the female castration complex. In E Jones (ed.) Selected Papers on Psycho-Analysis. London: Maresfield Reprints (1979), 338-69.

Abraham K (1921) Contribution to the theory of the anal character. In E Jones (ed.) Selected Papers on Psycho-Analysis. London: Maresfield Reprints (1979), 370-92.

Abraham K (1924) A short study of the development of the libido, viewed in the light of mental disorders. In E Jones (ed.) Selected Papers of Karl Abraham. London: Hogarth Press (1942), 418-501.

Arlow JA (1969a) Fantasy, memory and reality testing, Psychoanalytic Quarterly 38: 28-51.

Arlow JA (1969b) Unconscious fantasy and disturbances of conscious experience, Psychoanalytic Quarterly 38: 1-27.

Balint M (1968) The Basic Fault. London: Tavistock.

Baranger W (1971) Posicion y Objeto en la Obra de Melanie Klein. Buenos Aires: Ediciones Kargieman.

Baranger W (1980) Validez del concepto de objeto en la obra de Melanie Klein. In Aportaciones al Concepto de Objeto en Psicoanalisis. Buenos Aires: Amorrortu.

Bell D, Segal H (1991) The theory of narcissism in the work of Freud and Klein. In P Fonagy, J Sandler, E Person (eds), Freud's 'On Narcissism: An Introduction'. New Haven and London: Yale University Press, 149-74.

Beres D (1962) The unconscious fantasy, Psychoanalytic Quarterly 21: 309-28.

De Bianchedi ET, Antar R, De Podetti MR et al. (1984) Beyond Freudian metapsychology: the metapsychological points of view of the Kleinian School, International Journal of Psychoanalysis 65: 389-98.

Bion WR (1957a) Differentiation of the psychotic from the non-psychotic personalities, International Journal of Psychoanalysis 38: 266-75. Also in Second Thoughts. London: Heinemann Medical Books (1967) 73-64.

Bion WR (1957b) On arrogance. In Second Thoughts. London: Heinemann Medical Books (1967), 86-92.

Bion WR (1959) Attacks on linking, International Journal of Psychoanalysis 40: 308-15. In Second Thoughts. London: Heinemann Medical Books (1967), 93-109.

Bion WR (1962a) Learning from Experience. London: Heinemann.

Bion WR (1962b) A theory of thinking, International Journal of Psychoanalysis 43: 306-10. In Second Thoughts. London: Heinemann Medical Books (1967), 110-119.

Bion WR (1963) Elements of psycho-analysis. In Seven Servants. Northvale, New Jersey: Jason Aronson (1977), 1-109.

Bion WR (1970) Attention and Interpretation. London: Tavistock.

Bion WR (1992) Cogitations. London: Karnac.

Bleandonu G (1994) Wilfred Bion: His Life and Works 1907-1979. London: Free Association Books.

Bower TGR (1977) Le developpement psychologique de la première enfance. Brussels: Pierre Mardaga.

Brenman E (1985) Cruelty and narrow-mindedness, International Journal of Psychoanalysis 66: 273-82.

Britton R (1989) The missing link: parental sexuality in the Oedipus complex. In R Britton, M Feldman, E O'Shaughnessy, J Steiner (eds), The Oedipus Complex Today: Clinical Implications. London: Karnac, 83-102.

Britton R (1995) Reality and unreality in phantasy and fiction. In ES Person, P Fonagy, SA Figueira (eds), On Freud's 'Creative Writers and Day-Dreaming'. New Haven: Yale University Press.

Britton R (1998a) Belief and Imagination. London: Routledge.

Britton R (1998b) Contribution to panel discussion on 'The Controversial Discussions: Fifty Years Later'. Paper presented at the Fall 1998 Meeting of the American Psychoanalytic Association, New York. Unpublished.

Bronstein C (1997) Technique and interpretation in Klein. In B Burgoyne, M Sullivan (eds), The Klein-Lacan Dialogues. London: Rebus Press, 37-43.

Caper R (1988) Immaterial Facts. Northvale, New Jersey: Jason Aronson.

Carpenter CG (1975) Mother's face and the newborn. In R Lewin (ed.), Child Alive. London: Temple Smith.

Dante Alighieri (1954) La Divina Commedia. Verona: Arnoldo Mondadori.

Feldman M (1995) Grievance: the underlying Oedipal configuration. Paper presented at the March 1995 West Lodge Conference, West Lodge, Great Britain. Unpublished.

Feldman M (1997) Projective identification: the analyst's involvement, International Journal of Psychoanalysis 78: 227-45.

Ferenczi S (1909) Introjection and transference. In First Contributions to Psycho-Analysis Trans. E Jones. London: Karnac (1980), 35-93.

Ferenczi S (1912) On the definition of introjection. In M. Balint (ed.) Final Contributions to the Problems and Methods of Psycho-Analysis. Trans. E Jones. London: Maresfield Reprints (1955), 316-18.

Ferenczi S (1913) Stages in the development of the sense of reality. In First Contributions to Psycho-Analysis. Trans. E Jones. London: Karnac (1980), 213-44.

Ferenczi S, Rank O (1924) The Development of Psychoanalysis. New York & Washington: Nervous and Mental Disease Publishing Co.

Freud A (1937) The Ego and the Mechanisms of Defence. London: Hogarth Press.

Freud A (1966) Normality and Pathology in Childhood. London: Hogarth Press.

Freud S (1895) Extracts from Fliess papers: Draft H. In J Strachey (ed.), The Standard Edition of the Complete Psychological Works of Sigmund Freud (vol. 1). London: Hogarth Press, 206-13.

Freud S (1896) Further remarks on the neuro-psychosis of defence. In J Strachey (ed.), The Standard Edition of the Complete Psychological Works of Sigmund Freud (vol. 3). London: Hogarth Press, 157-85.

Freud S (1900) The interpretation of dreams. In J Strachey (ed.), The Standard Edition of the Complete Psychological Works of Sigmund Freud (vols 4 and 5). London: Hogarth Press, 1-715.

Freud S (1901) The psychopathology of everyday life. In J Strachey (ed.), The Standard Edition of the Complete Psychological Works of Sigmund Freud (vol. 6). London: Hogarth Press, 1-190.

Freud S (1905a) Fragment of an analysis of a case of hysteria. In J Strachey (ed.), The Standard Edition of the Complete Psychological Works of Sigmund Freud (vol. 7). London: Hogarth Press, 7-122.

Freud S (1905b) Three essays on the theory of sexuality. In J Strachey (ed.), The Standard Edition of the Complete Psychological Works of Sigmund Freud (vol. 7). London: Hogarth Press, 123-230.

Freud S (1908) Hysterical phantasies and their relation to bisexuality. In J. Stratchey (ed.), The Standard Edition of the Complete Psychological Works of Sigmund Freud (vol. 9). London: Hogarth, 159-66.

Freud S (1910a) Leonardo Da Vinci and a memory of his childhood. In J Strachey (ed.), The Standard Edition of the Complete Psychological Works of Sigmund Freud (vol. 11). London: Hogarth Press, 57-137.

Freud S (1910b) A special type of choice of object made by men. In J Strachey (ed.), The Standard Edition of the Complete Psychological Works of Sigmund Freud (vol. 11). London: Hogarth Press, 164-75.

Freud S (1911a) Formulations on the two principles of mental functioning. In J Strachey (ed.), The Standard Edition of the Complete Psychological Works of Sigmund Freud (vol. 12). London: Hogarth Press (1958-78), 67-104.

Freud S (1911b) Psycho-analytic notes upon an autobiographical account of a case of paranoia (Dementia Paranoides). In J Strachey (ed.), The Standard Edition of the Complete Psychological Works of Sigmund Freud (vol. 12). London: Hogarth Press (1958-78).

Freud S (1914) On narcissism: an introduction. In J Strachey (ed.), The Standard Edition of the Complete Psychological Works of Sigmund Freud (vol. 14). London: Hogarth Press, 67-104.

Freud S (1915a) Instincts and their vicissitudes. In J Strachey (ed.), The Standard Edition of the Complete Psychological Works of Sigmund Freud (vol. 14). London: Hogarth Press, 109-40.

Freud S (1915b) Observations on transference love: further recommendations on the technique of psycho-analysis. In J Strachey (ed.), The Standard Edition of the Complete Psychological Works of Sigmund Freud (vol. 12). London: Hogarth Press, 157-71.

Freud S (1915c) Repression. In J Strachey (ed.), The St`andard Edition of the Complete Psychological Works of Sigmund Freud (vol. 14). London: Hogarth Press, 141-58.

Freud S (1915d) The unconscious. In J Strachey (ed.), The Standard Edition of the Complete Psychological Works of Sigmund Freud (vol. 14). London: Hogarth Press, 159-215.

Freud S (1916-17) The paths to the formation of symptoms. Lecture XXIII in Introductory Lectures on Psycho-Analysis. In J Strachey (ed.) The Standard Edition of the Complete Psychological Works of Sigmund Freud (vol. 17). London: Hogarth Press, 358-77.

Freud S (1917) Mourning and melancholia. In J Strachey (ed.), The Standard Edition of the Complete Psychological Works of Sigmund Freud (vol. 14). London: Hogarth Press, 237–58.

Freud S (1917) On transformations of instinct as exemplified in anal eroticism. In J Strachey (ed.) The Standard Edition of the Complete Psychological Works of Sigmund Freud (vol. 17). London: Hogarth Press, 127–33.

Freud S (1920a) Beyond the pleasure principle. In J Strachey (ed.), The Standard Edition of the Complete Psychological Works of Sigmund Freud (vol. 18). London: Hogarth Press, 1–64.

Freud S (1920b) From the history of an infantile neurosis. In J Strachey (ed.), The Standard Edition of the Complete Psychological Works of Sigmund Freud (vol. 17). London: Hogarth Press, 3–122.

Freud S (1921) Group psychology and the analysis of the ego. In J Strachey (ed.), The Standard Edition of the Complete Psychological Works of Sigmund Freud (vol. 18). London: Hogarth Press, 69–143.

Freud S (1923) The ego and the id. In J Strachey (ed.), The Standard Edition of the Complete Psychological Works of Sigmund Freud (vol. 19). London: Hogarth Press, 1–59.

Freud S (1924) The dissolution of the Oedipus complex. In J Strachey (ed.), The Standard Edition of the Complete Psychological Works of Sigmund Freud (vol. 19). London: Hogarth Press, 173–82.

Freud S (1933) New introductory lectures on psychoanalysis. In J Strachey (ed.), The Standard Edition of the Complete Psychological Works of Sigmund Freud (vol. 22). London: Hogarth Press, 1–182.

Freud S (1937) Analysis terminable and interminable. In J Strachey (ed.), The Standard Edition of the Complete Psychological Works of Sigmund Freud (vol. 23). London: Hogarth Press, 209–53.

Freud S (1938) An outline of psychoanalysis. In J Strachey (ed.), The Standard Edition of the Complete Psychological Works of Sigmund Freud (vol. 23). London: Hogarth Press, 139–208.

Freud S (1940) Splitting of the ego in the process of defence. In J Strachey (ed.), The Standard Edition of the Complete Psychological Works of Sigmund Freud (vol. 23). London: Hogarth Press, 275–8.

Grosskurth P (1986) Melanie Klein. London: Maresfield Library.

Harris MH (1976) The contribution of observation of mother–infant interaction and development to the equipment of a psychoanalyst or psychoanalytic psychotherapist. In MH Williams (ed.), Collected Papers of Martha Harris and Esther Bick. Strathtay: Clunie Press, 225–39.

Hayman A (1989) What do we mean by 'phantasy'?, International Journal of Psychoanalysis 70: 105–14.

Heimann P (1942) 'A contribution to the problem of sublimation and its relation to processes of internalization.' International Journal of Psychoanalysis 23, 8–17. Also in About Children and Children-No-Longer. M. Tonnesmann. The New Library of Psychoanalysis. Routledge 1989, 26–45.

Heimann P (1950) On countertransference, International Journal of Psychoanalysis 31: 81–4.

Heimann P, Isaacs S (1952) Regression. In J Riviere (ed.), Developments in Psycho-Analysis. London: Hogarth Press. 169–97.

Hinshelwood RD (1989) A Dictionary of Kleinian Thought. London: Free Association Books.

Hinshelwood RD (1997) The elusive concept of 'internal objects' (1934-1943): its role in the formation of the Klein Group, International Journal of Psychoanalysis 78: 877-97.

Hug-Hellmuth H (1921) On the technique of child analysis. International Journal of Psychoanalysis 2: 287-303.

Isaacs S (1948) The nature and function of phantasy. International Journal of Psychoanalysis 29: 73-97. In M Klein, P Heimann, S Isaacs, J Riviere (eds), Developments in Psycho-Analysis. London: Hogarth Press (1952), 67-121.

Jacques E (1965) Death and the midlife crisis, International Journal of Psychoanalysis 46: 502-14.

James H (1888) The Aspern Papers in 'The New York edition of the Novels and Tales of Henny James'. New York: Scnibner 1907-9.

Joffe WG (1969) A critical review of the status of the envy concept, International Journal of Psychoanalysis 50: 533-45.

Jones E (1916) The theory of symbolism. In Papers on Psycho-Analysis. London: Maresfield Reprints (1977), 87-144.

Joseph B (1981) Defence mechanisms and phantasy in the psychoanalytic process. In M Feldman, EB Spillius (eds), Psychic Equilibrium and Psychic Change: Selected Papers of Betty Joseph. London: Routledge (1989), 116-26.

Joseph B (1985) Transference: the total situation, International Journal of Psychoanalysis 66: 447-54. Reprinted in Melanie Klein Today, Vol. 2. London: Routledge (1988), 61-72.

Joseph B (1989) Psychic Equilibrium and Psychic Change. London: Routledge.

Joseph B (1998) Thinking about a playroom, Journal of Child Psychotherapy 24: 359-66.

King P, Steiner R (eds) (1991) The Freud-Klein Controversies: 1941-45. London: Routledge.

Klein M (1921) The development of a child. In Love, Guilt and Reparation and Other Works 1921-1945: The Writings of Melanie Klein, Volume I. London: Hogarth Press (1975), 1-53.

Klein M (1923a) Early analysis. In Love, Guilt and Reparation and Other Works 1921-1945: The Writings of Melanie Klein, Volume I. London: Hogarth Press (1975), 77-105.

Klein M (1923b) The role of the school in the libidinal development of the child. In Love, Guilt and Reparation and Other Works 1921-1945: The Writings of Melanie Klein, Volume I. London: Hogarth Press (1975), 59-76.

Klein M (1925) A contribution to the psychogenesis of tics. In Love, Guilt and Reparation and Other Works 1921-1945: The Writings of Melanie Klein, Volume I. London: Hogarth Press (1975), 106-27.

Klein M (1926) The psychological principles of early analysis. In Love, Guilt and Reparation and Other Works 1921-1945: The Writings of Melanie Klein, Volume I. London: Hogarth Press (1975), 128-38.

Klein M (1927) Symposium on child analysis. In Love, Guilt and Reparation and Other Works 1921-1945: The Writings of Melanie Klein, Volume I. London: Hogarth Press (1975), 139-69.

Klein M (1928) Early stages of the Oedipus complex. In Love, Guilt and Reparation and Other Works 1921-1945: The Writings of Melanie Klein, Volume I. London: Hogarth Press (1975), 186-98.

Klein M (1929) Infantile anxiety-situations reflected in a work of art and in the creative impulse. In Love, Guilt and Reparation and Other Works 1921-1945: The Writings of Melanie Klein, Volume I. London: Hogarth Press (1975), 210-17.

Klein M (1930) The importance of symbol-formation in the development of the ego. In Love, Guilt and Reparation and Other Works 1921-1945: The Writings of Melanie Klein, Volume I. London: Hogarth Press (1975), 219-32.

Klein M (1932) The psycho-analysis of children: The Writings of Melanie Klein Volume II. London: Hogarth Press (1975).

Klein M (1933) The early development of conscience in the child. In Love, Guilt and Reparation and Other Works 1921-1945: The Writings of Melanie Klein, Volume I. London: Hogarth Press (1975), 248-57

Klein M (1935) A contribution to the psychogenesis of manic-depressive states. In Love, Guilt and Reparation and Other Works 1921-1945: The Writings of Melanie Klein, Volume I. London: Hogarth Press (1975), 236-89.

Klein M (1936) Weaning. In Love, Guilt and Reparation and Other Works 1921-1945: The Writings of Melanie Klein, Volume I. London: Hogarth Press (1975), 290-305.

Klein M (1940) Mourning and its relation to manic-depressive states. In Love, Guilt and Reparation and Other Works 1921-1945: The Writings of Melanie Klein, Volume I. London: Hogarth Press (1975), 344-69.

Klein M (1945) The Oedipus complex in the light of early anxieties. In Love, Guilt and Reparation and Other Works 1921-1945: The Writings of Melanie Klein, Volume I. London: Hogarth Press (1975), 370-419.

Klein M (1946) Notes on some schizoid mechanisms, IJPA 27: 99-110; also appears (with slight differences in each case) in the following: (a) IJPA 27: 99-110; (b) J Riviere (ed.), Developments in Psychoanalysis [1952]. London: Karnac Books (1989), 292-320; (c) Envy and Gratitude and Other Works 1946-1963: The Writings of Melanie Klein, Volume III. London: Hogarth Press (1975), 292-320.

Klein M (1948) On the theory of anxiety and guilt. In Envy and Gratitude and Other Works 1946-1963: The Writings of Melanie Klein, Volume III. London: Hogarth Press (1975), 25-42.

Klein M (1952a) The mutual influences in the development of ego and id. In Envy and Gratitude and Other Works 1946-1963: The Writings of Melanie Klein, Volume III. London: Hogarth Press (1975), 57-60.

Klein M (1952b) The origins of transference. In Envy and Gratitude and Other Works 1946-1963: The Writings of Melanie Klein, Volume III. London: Hogarth Press (1975), 48-56.

Klein M (1952c) Some theoretical conclusions regarding the emotional life of the infant. In Developments in Psychoanalysis. London: Karnac (1989), 198-236; also appears in Envy and Gratitude and Other Works 1946-1963: The Writings of Melanie Klein, Volume III. London: Hogarth Press (1975), 61-93.

Klein M (1955a) On identification. In Envy and Gratitude and Other Works 1946-1963: The Writings of Melanie Klein, Volume III. London: Hogarth Press (1975), 141-75.

Klein, M (1955b) The psycho-analytic play technique: its history and significance. In Envy and Gratitude and Other Works 1946-1963: The Writings of Melanie Klein, Volume III. London: Hogarth Press (1975), 122-40.

Klein M (1957) Envy and gratitude. In Envy and Gratitude and Other Works 1946-1963: The Writings of Melanie Klein, Volume III. London: Hogarth Press (1975), 176-235.

Klein M (1958) On the development of mental functioning. In Envy and Gratitude and Other Works 1946-1963: The Writings of Melanie Klein, Volume III. London: Hogarth Press, 1975, 236-46.

Klein M (1959a) Autobiography, unpublished, Wellcome Trust.

Klein M (1959b) Our adult world and its roots in infancy. In Envy and Gratitude and Other Works 1946-1963: The Writings of Melanie Klein, Volume III. London: Hogarth Press (1975), 247-63.

Klein M (1975a) Love, Guilt and Reparation and Other Works 1921-1945: The Writings of Melanie Klein, Volume I. London: Hogarth Press.

Klein M (1975b) Envy and Gratitude and Other Works 1946-1963: The Writings of Melanie Klein, Volume III. London: Hogarth Press.

Kris E (1935) The psychology of caricature. In Psychoanalytic Exploration in Art. New York: International Universities Press (1952).

Kristeva J (2000) Le genie feminin. Tome II: Melanie Klein. Paris: Editions Fayard.

Laplanche J (1981) The Unconscious and the Id. London: Rebus Press (1999).

Laplanche J, Pontalis J-B (1973) The Language of Psychoanalysis. London: Hogarth Press, 314-19.

Malcolm R (1999) On Bearing Unbearable States of Mind. The New Library of Psychoanalysis, Priscilla Roth (ed.) London: Routledge.

Meltzer D (1966) The relation of anal masturbation to projective identification, International Journal of Psychoanalysis 47: 335-42; also appears in EB Spillius (ed.), Melanie Klein Today. London: The New Library of Psychoanalysis; New York: Routledge (1988), 102-16.

Meltzer D (1978) The Kleinian Development. Strathtay: Clunie Press.

Merea EC (1980) Los conceptos de objeto en la obra de Freud. In W Baranger (ed.), Aportaciones al Concerpto de Objeto en Psicoanalisis. Buenos Aires: Amorrortu, 3-22.

Milton J (1975) Paradise Lost. New York: Norton.

Mitchell J (1991) The Selected Melanie Klein. London: Penguin.

Money-Kyrle R (1968) Cognitive development, International Journal of Psychoanalysis 49: 691-8.

O'Shaughnessy E (1999) Relating to the superego, International Journal of Psychoanalysis 80: 861-70.

Petot J-M (1979) Melanie Klein, Premieres Decouvertes et Premier Systeme 1919-1932 (vol. 1). Paris: Dunod.

Petot J-M (1982) Melanie Klein, Le Moi et le Bon Object 1932-1960 (vol. 2). Paris: Dunod.

Petot J-M (1990) Melanie Klein, First Discoveries and First System 1919-1932 (vol. 1). Madison, CT: International Universities Press.

Petot J-M (1991) Melanie Klein, The Ego and the Good Object, 1932-1960 (vol. 2). Madison, CT: International Universities Press.

Polkinghorne JC (1986) The Quantum World. London: Penguin.

Proust M (1981) Remembrance of Things Past. London: Chatto & Windus.

Racker H (1968) Transference and Countertransference. London: Hogarth Press.

Riesenberg-Malcolm R (1981) Expiation as a defence, International Journal of Psychoanalytic Psychotherapy 8: 549-70.

Riesenberg-Malcolm R (1999) The constitution and operation of the super-ego. In P Roth (ed.) On Bearing Unbearable States of Mind. London: Routledge, 53-70.

Riviere J (1936) A contribution to the analysis of the negative therapeutic reaction, International Journal of Psychoanalysis 17: 304-20.

Rosenfeld H (1950) Notes on the psychopathology of confusional states in chronic schizophrenia, International Journal of Psychoanalysis 31: 132-7.

Rosenfeld H (1952) Notes on the psycho-analysis of the superego conflict in an acute schizophrenic patient, International Journal of Psycho-Analysis 33: 111-31. Also appears in Psychotic States: A Psycho-Analytical Approach. London: Maresfield Reprints; New York: International Universities Press (1965), 63-103,

Rosenfeld H (1964) An investigation into the need of neurotic and psychotic patients to act out during analysis. In Psychotic States: A Psycho-Analytical Approach. New York: International Universities Press (1965), 200-16.

Rosenfeld H (1971a) A clinical approach to the psychoanalytic theory of the life and death instincts: an investigation into the aggressive aspects of narcissism, International Journal of Psychoanalysis 52: 169-78.

Rosenfeld H (1971b) Contribution to the psychopathology of psychotic states: the importance of projective identification in the ego structure and the object relations of the psychotic patient. In P Doucet, C Laurin (eds), Problems of Psychosis. The Hague: Excerpta Medica, 115-28; also appears in EB Spillius (ed.), Melanie Klein Today (vol. 1). London: The New Library of Psychoanalysis; New York: Routledge (1988), 117-37.

Rosenfeld H (1978) Notes on the psychopathology and psychoanalytic treatment of some borderline patients, International Journal of Psychoanalysis 59: 215-21.

Rosenfeld H (1983) Primitive object relations and mechanisms, International Journal of Psychoanalysis 64: 261-7.

Rosenfeld H (1987a) Impasse and Interpretation. London: Tavistock Publications.

Rosenfeld H (1987b) Narcissistic patients with negative therapeutic reactions. In Impasse and Interpretation. London: Tavistock Publications, 85-104.

Rustin M (1997) Child psychotherapy within the Kleinian tradition. In B Burgoyne, M Sullivan (eds), The Klein-Lacan Dialogues. London: Rebus Press, 7-17.

Rycroft C (1968) Phantasy. In A Critical Dictionary of Psychoanalysis. London: Nelson, 118.

Sander LW (1969) Regulation and organization in the early infant-caretaker system. In RJ Robinson et al. (eds), Brain and Early Behavior. London: Academic Press.

Sandler J (1976a) Countertransference and role-responsiveness, International Review of Psycho-Analysis 3: 43-7.

Sandler J (1976b) Dreams, unconscious phantasies, and 'identity of perception', International Review of Psycho-Analysis 3: 33-42.

Sandler J (1983) Reflections on some relations between psychoanalytic concepts and psychoanalytic practice, International Journal of Psychoanalysis 64: 35-45.

Sandler J (1987) Projection, Identification, Projective Identification. London: Karnac Books.

Sandler J, Nagera H (1963) Aspects of the metapsychology of fantasy, Psychoanalytic Study of the Child 18: 159-94.

Sandler J, Sandler A-M (1983) The 'second censorship', the 'three-box model', and some technical implications, International Journal of Psychoanalysis 64: 413-26.

Sandler, J, Sandler, A-M (1984) The past unconscious, the present unconscious, and interpretation of the transference, Psychoanalytic Inquiry 4: 367-99.

Sandler J, Sandler A-M (1986) The gyroscopic function of unconscious fantasy. In DB Feinsilver (ed.), Towards a Comprehensive Model for Schizophrenic Disorders. New York: Analytic Press, 109-23.

Sandler J, Sandler A-M (1987) The past unconscious, the present unconscious and the vicissitudes of guilt, International Journal of Psychoanalysis 68: 331-41.

Sandler J, Sandler A-M (1998) A theory of internal object relations. In Internal Objects

Revisited. London: Karnac, 121-40.

Sandler J, Holder A, Dare C (1972-82) Frames of reference in psychoanalytic psychology. I-XII, British Journal of Medical Psychology 45-9, 51, 55.

Sandler J, Dare C, Holder A, Deher AU (1997) Freud's Models of the Mind: An Introduction. London: Karnac.

Schafer R (1997) The Contemporary Kleinians of London. Madison, Connecticut: International Universities Press.

Segal H (1950) Some aspects of the analysis of a schizophrenic, International Journal of Psychoanalysis 31: 268-78.

Segal H (1952) A psycho-analytical approach to aesthetics, International Journal of Psychoanalysis 33: 196-207.

Segal H (1957) Notes on symbol formation. In The Work of Hanna Segal. Northvale, New Jersey: Jason Aronson (1981), 49-65.

Segal H (1964) Phantasy and other processes. In The Work of Hanna Segal. Northvale, New Jersey: Jason Aronson (1981), 41-7.

Segal H (1967) Melanie Klein's technique. In The Work of Hanna Segal. Northvale, New Jersey: Jason Aronson (1981), 3-24.

Segal H (1973) Introduction to the Work of Melanie Klein. London: Hogarth Press.

Segal H (1978) On symbolism. International Journal of Psychoanalysis 59: 315-19.

Segal H (1979) Klein. London: Fontana Modern Masters.

Segal H (1980) Melanie Klein. New York: Viking Press.

Segal H (1990) Dream, Phantasy and Art. London: Routledge.

Segal H (1993) On the clinical usefulness of the concept of the death instinct, International Journal of Psychoanalysis 74: 55-61.

Segal H (1997a) From Hiroshima to the Gulf War and after: socio-political expressions of ambivalence. In J Steiner (ed.), Psychoanalysis, Literature and War. London: Routledge, 157-68.

Segal H (1997b) Psychoanalysis, Literature and War. London: Routledge.

Segal H (1999) What is an object? The role of perception. In P Fonagy, A Cooper, R Wallerstein (eds), Psychoanalysis On the Move: The Work of Joseph Sandler. London: New Library of Psychoanalysis.

Shakespeare W (1969) Othello. London: Penguin.

Sohn L (1985) Narcissistic organisation, projective identification and the formation of the identificate, International Journal of Psychoanalysis 66: 201-13.

Spillius EB (1988a) Melanie Klein Today: Developments in Theory and Practice. Volume I: Mainly Theory. London: Routledge.

Spillius EB (1988b) Melanie Klein Today: Developments in Theory and Practice. Volume II: Mainly Practice. London: Routledge.

Spillius EB (1993) Varieties of envious experiences, International Journal of Psychoanalysis 74: 1199-212.

Spillius EB (1994) Developments in Kleinian thought: overview and personal view. Psychoanalytic Inquiry 14: 324-64.

Steiner J (1985) Turning a blind eye: the cover up for Oedipus, International Review of Psychoanalysis 12: 161-72.

Steiner J (1987) The interplay between pathological organisations and the paranoid-schizoid and depressive positions, International Journal of Psychoanalysis 68: 69-80.

Steiner J (1993) Psychic retreats: Pathological organisations in psychotic, neurotic and borderline patients. London: Routledge.

Steiner R (1988) Paths to Xanadu ... some notes on the development of dream displacement and condensation in Sigmund Freud's Interpretation of Dreams, International Review of Psychoanalysis 15: 415-54.

Stonebridge L, Phillips J (1998) Reading Melanie Klein. London: Routledge.

Strachey J (1934) The nature of the therapeutic action of psychoanalysis, International Journal of Psychoanalysis 15: 127-59.

Styron W (1991) Darkness Visible. London: Picador.

Weil J (1964) Life with a Star. London: Collins (1989).

Winnicott DW (1954) Metapsychological and clinical aspects of regression within the psycho-analytical set-up. In Through Paediatrics to Psycho-Analysis. London: Hogarth Press (1975), 278-329.

Winnicott DW (1960) The theory of the parent-infant relationship. In J Sutherland (ed.) The Maturational Process and the Facilitating Environment. London: Hogarth Press (1976), 37-55.

Wollheim R (1969) The mind and the mind's image of itself, International Journal of Psychoanalysis 50: 209-20.

Index